PANDEMIC BIOETHICS

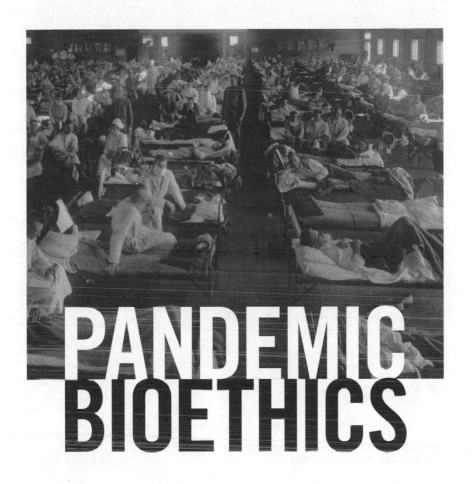

PANDEMIC
BIOETHICS

GREGORY E. PENCE

broadview press

BROADVIEW PRESS – www.broadviewpress.com
Peterborough, Ontario, Canada

Founded in 1985, Broadview Press remains a wholly independent publishing house. Broadview's focus is on academic publishing; our titles are accessible to university and college students as well as scholars and general readers. With 800 titles in print, Broadview has become a leading international publisher in the humanities, with world-wide distribution. Broadview is committed to environmentally responsible publishing and fair business practices.

Library and Archives Canada Cataloguing in Publication

Title: Pandemic bioethics / Gregory E. Pence.
Names: Pence, Gregory E., author.
Description: Includes bibliographical references and index.
Identifiers: Canadiana (print) 20210205490 | Canadiana (ebook) 20210205644 | ISBN
    9781554815210 (softcover) | ISBN 9781770488090 (PDF) | ISBN 9781460407585 (EPUB)
Subjects: LCSH: Epidemiology—Moral and ethical aspects. | LCSH: Medical ethics. | LCSH: Public
    health—Moral and ethical aspects. | LCSH: Bioethics.
Classification: LCC RA652 .P46 2021 | DDC 174.2/944—dc23

Broadview Press handles its own distribution in North America:
PO Box 1243, Peterborough, Ontario K9J 7H5, Canada
555 Riverwalk Parkway, Tonawanda, NY 14150, USA
Tel: (705) 743-8990; Fax: (705) 743-8353
email: customerservice@broadviewpress.com

For all territories outside of North America, distribution is handled by Eurospan Group.

Broadview Press acknowledges the financial support of the Government of Canada for our publishing activities.

Canadä

Edited by Martin R. Boyne

Book design by Chris Rowat Design

PRINTED IN CANADA

CONTENTS

PREFACE

Nearly 50 years ago, bioethics captivated me when I first published a note in the *Hastings Center Report*. Since then, bioethics has become the most intellectually exciting field in academia today. When China locked down 46 million citizens in Wuhan in December 2019, I knew that bioethics had just met the biggest issue of its modern life. This book explores the many ethical issues raised by this new pandemic.

Of course, pandemics have hurt humans before, and previous mistakes in confronting pandemics are worth learning, lest we repeat those errors. This book's first two chapters review that history. Good bioethics also builds on good facts, so the next chapter explores what we know about viruses in general and SARS-CoV-2 in particular. After that, the fourth chapter discusses four approaches that governments around the world used to confront the coronavirus, with varying results and philosophical assumptions. Several issues emerge in many chapters: just distribution (of ventilators, vaccines, harms of lockdowns), vaccine passports, rollout of vaccines, leadership, and trade-offs between saving lives in the ICU versus saving the economy.

Ethical theory and philosophical tools can illuminate issues arising from pandemics, and for me, the best approach to them is not top-down but bottom-up, using theories that emerge in a specific context, for example, utilitarianism in discussing allocation of vaccines, or using a particular concept, such as the Trolley Problem, to offer new insights. In my career, I've often been amazed at how, when I drill down deep into a complex case, new ethical issues appear that I hadn't seen at the start, such as those that emerge about immunity passports. Philosophical perspectives also arise when discussing the four general approaches to the pandemic by countries as different as Canada and Niger.

Of course, it is easy to look back a year and see the mistakes that were made, but in the midst of life-and-death decisions, no such ease can be had. Anyone writing about pandemic ethics should do so with a large amount of humility, knowing how easy it is to get facts wrong, miss important issues, or incorrectly anticipate consequences. Any mistakes of that nature are mine alone, but I hope that readers will, by the end of the book, understand that we all must fight pandemics together.

NOTES TO THE READER

For convenience in this book, the medical condition COVID-19 is written simply as "Covid," and the virus SARS CoV-2 is written as "SARS2."

Every effort has been made to make this book as accurate as possible, but the world's knowledge of SARS2 and its variants is evolving quickly. Please email the author (pence@uab.edu) about any topic that needs to be updated or clarified and future editions of this text will address those concerns.

CHAPTER 1
HISTORICAL EPIDEMICS

The great English science journalist Laura Spinney wrote one of the definitive accounts of the Spanish flu of 1918, a book that was little read until the coronavirus appeared in 2020. In *Pale Rider: The Spanish Flu of 1918 and How It Changed the World*, she introduced her subject thus:

> The Spanish flu infected one in three people on earth, or 500 million human beings. Between the first case recorded on 4 March 1918, and the last sometime in March 1920, it killed 50–100 million people, or between 2.5 and 5 percent of the global population—a range that reflects the uncertainty that still surrounds it. In terms of single events causing major loss of life, it surpassed the First World War (17 million dead), the Second World War (60 million dead) and possibly both put together It was the greatest tidal wave of death since the Black Death, perhaps of human history.[1]

As philosopher George Santayana famously observed, "Those who are ignorant of history are condemned to repeat its mistakes." We cannot undo history, but we can learn from it. We can learn from the mistakes of past societies that confronted pandemics such as the Spanish flu that Spinney discusses. Maybe we can even learn how to prepare for future pandemics.

This chapter addresses historical pandemics and their bioethical issues, including plague, cholera, malaria, smallpox, and the Spanish flu of 1918. In the next chapter, we examine more modern pandemics, especially those caused by viruses such as polio and Ebola.

When an infectious disease affects only one region, it's an *epidemic*, but when it spreads to several continents, it's a *pandemic*. Pandemics are not new in human history, yet as Albert Camus wrote in *The Plague*, "Everybody knows that pestilences have a way of recurring in the world, yet somehow we find it hard to believe in ones that crash down on our heads from a blue sky. There have been as many plagues as wars in history, yet always plagues and wars take people equally by surprise."[2] The Spanish flu pandemic—which actually began in Kansas and not in Spain—quickly spread to Europe during World War I and then to every inhabited continent.[3]

Overall, germs don't care whether we accept them or not; they don't care about who is virtuous or who is vicious, who deserves to die and who doesn't, who looks clean and who looks dirty. When then-president Donald Trump invited guests to the Rose Garden of the White House in September 2020, SARS2 hitched a ride and did not distinguish between the famous and the anonymous. Viruses just want hosts to use to replicate themselves. The recent novel *Where the Crawdads Sing* expresses this idea well: "judgement had no place here. Evil was not in play, just life pulsing on, even at the expense of some of the players. Biology sees Right and Wrong as the same color in different light."[4]

THE SPANISH FLU OF 1918

In interesting ways, the pandemic of the Spanish flu of 1918 presaged today's Covid pandemic. (Because everyone refers to this flu as "the Spanish flu of 1918," I will also do so.) It began in the spring of 1918, lessened in harm during that summer as it traveled around the globe, and returned with a vengeance in the late fall, probably with a variant of the original virus, killing more in three months then than it had previously. Similarly, in March 2020, SARS2 killed the most in Britain, and in April hospitalized many, becoming less harmful over the summer, and then created a deadly second wave in late December, when it hospitalized over 20,000, pushing the National Health Service to its limit.

This Spanish flu scared North Americans. People got sick one morning and died the next. Because those hospitalized often died for lack of oxygen, their skin turned dark and, as they died, a bloody froth erupted from their noses and mouths. Doctors looking down rows of patients lying on beds in big hospital wards couldn't distinguish white from black patients. The Spanish flu lasted two years, infected perhaps 500 million people, and killed at least 50 million of them. It probably killed twice that number, but no one kept statistics for remote parts of Africa, South America, or Asia, so that is an epistemic black hole. (A milder variant continued for another six months in 1920, but it only seemed like a bad flu.[5])

Some cities acted stupidly with Spanish flu. On October 20, 1918, the premiere of Charlie Chaplin's film *Shoulder Arms* opened to a packed crowd in Manhattan, where the manager congratulated the crowd for coming out. Several days later, this manager died of flu.[6] As the historian John Barry explains in his classic *The Great Influenza: The Story of the Deadliest Pandemic in History*, when a British merchant ship unloaded at the Navy Yard in Philadelphia, the Spanish flu entered the city.[7] Within days, and by September 15, 600 sailors were hospitalized.[8] Its public health officer, Dr. Wilmer Krusen, faced pressure to minimize the lethality of the new virus. After a few sailors had died, he was forced to say that the Spanish flu amounted to nothing more than "old-fashioned influenza," a terrible lie, one that would kill many Philadelphians. Worse, Dr. Krusen agreed with city leaders not to confine sailors to the Navy Yard, so they drank and caroused at bars downtown.

On September 28, Philadelphia's mayor ignored advice from scientists, who advised him that citizens should avoid large gatherings. Instead, he held the largest parade in the city's history, the Liberty Loan Parade, designed to stir patriotic fervor and get citizens to buy war bonds. One-ninth of the city's population of 2 million turned out, packed 15-deep along sidewalks.[9] Within days, the virus struck hundreds of policemen. During just one week in October, 4,500 Philadelphians died, 837 on just one day.[10] By the time the killer virus had cut through the city, 150,000 citizens had been infected and 17,500 had died, one of the highest rates of both infection and death from Spanish flu anywhere in the world.[11] *Amplification systems* allow viruses to spread not just from one person to another but exponentially, from one person to dozens to hundreds to thousands. The Liberty Loan Parade illustrated such an amplification system, but many other things can be amplification systems for viruses: a community's blood bank, an interstate system, sharing needles and syringes, and international air travel.

When the Spanish flu first hit Kansas and started its lethal toll, the American press did not want to depress its readers, many of whom opposed their country's participation in the deadly, far-off World War I in Europe. When the new flu devasted soldiers and civilians in the fall of 1918, just when the war was ending, the press continued to suppress what the flu did, lest Americans lag in their support. By the time this flu had run its course over two years and killed 50 million, World War I was over, soldiers returned, and everybody moved on, beginning the Roaring Twenties.

Strangely, this virus attacked mainly those under age 40. Why? One theory hypothesized that seniors had previously been exposed to a deadly flu and had acquired immunity to future flus, but then decades had passed without a similar flu, making 1918's young people "flu virgins."[12] Another theory is that the Spanish flu killed the young by causing *cytokine storms*, where their young immune systems overreacted to the virus, creating extreme inflammation and throwing everything at the virus, even to the point of destroying the host's organs.

Importantly, such cytokine storms seem to be involved in 2020 in many of those hospitalized for Covid (I will say more about such storms in Chapter 3).

Of great importance for public health, authorities knew in 1918 that wearing masks, physical distancing, and avoiding large gatherings reduced the virus's spread and saved lives. Indeed, we can contrast efforts by successful and unsuccessful cities in containing this flu. A summary in 2007 in *Proceedings of the National Academy of Sciences* identified two key factors of cities that were successful in combating the Spanish flu:

(1) When the first cases hit, they quickly mandated lockdowns—they banned large gatherings, shuttered schools and businesses, and instituted physical distancing and even mask-wearing.

(2) After lockdowns, they did not re-open early.[13]

In his informative *Epidemics: The Impact of Germs and Their Power over Humanity*, Joshua Loomis, a microbiologist and historian, emphasizes that when cities lifted these restrictions too early, it "gave people a false sense of security at a time when the pandemic was still raging."[14] Of importance to Covid today, the virus spread quickly in cities where officials contradicted each other.[15] We can add to the conclusions of the above *Proceedings* a third fact about cities that were successful in curbing the virus:

(3) Successful cities issued consistent, evidence-based messages to the public about what to do. They did not conceal facts about the virus, change the facts, or pretend it wasn't deadly. They did not politicize facts about it.

What happened on college campuses and with sports in 1918 is fascinating. The United States declared war on Germany in April 1917, and the first recorded case of Spanish flu occurred on March 4, 1918. During the later fall of 1918, most college campuses contained boot camps to train soldiers, and many of them had football teams. At first, college presidents cancelled football, citing it as a distraction to military training. However, like the PAC 10 and Big 10 football conferences in 2020, presidents soon reversed their decisions, arguing that young men had too much time on their hands and that the public needed something to cheer about.[16] One football player finished his first game in Ohio and died 11 days later, while others in Texas and West Virginia died that fall. During that fall, almost 700 members of the University of Pittsburgh's Army training corps entered hospitals with the flu, and a hundred with pneumonia died.[17] Nevertheless, the team played on, tying for the national championship with Michigan.

In Katherine Ann Porter's *Pale Horse, Pale Rider*, her semi-autobiographical novella about two young lovers living during the Spanish flu, Miranda remarks, "It seems to be a plague, something out of the Middle Ages. Did you ever see so many funerals, ever?"[18] Porter herself became so ill with Spanish flu that she planned her own funeral.[19] This flu also hit Native Americans hard. In the Four Corners area of the American Southwest, over 3,000 people died. Entire Inuit villages died in Alaska.[20] However, despite the seriousness of this flu, we must remember that most infected people did not die. Of the 500 million people infected worldwide, if 50 million died, 90 percent survived. In the United States, about 550,000 died, so the Spanish flu killed only about one-half of 1 percent of the 100 million Americans then living, and 99.5 percent of Americans survived.[21]

The Spanish flu also differed from SARS2 in killing faster. According to historian John Barry, it did its worst damage in a particular geographical area, not gradually over years but often in only 15 weeks.[22] And afterwards, as Laura Spinney told National Public Radio in 2020, "humanity quickly bounces back...in the 1920s, there was a baby boom. And one of the reasons for that boom...is that the Spanish flu basically purged the world of people who were already sick with other diseases, notably tuberculosis. And so, what it left behind was a smaller but healthier population."[23]

CHOLERA

Cholera is caused by a bacterium, *Vibrio cholerae*, that thrives in warm water infected with fecal matter. The United States experienced a few epidemics of cholera during the nineteenth century, but Europe and Asia had seen them over thousands of years. Pilgrimages to Mecca and Medina in 1831 created amplification systems for cholera, killing at least 10,000 pilgrims and sickening many others; pilgrims who returned to Cairo and Alexandria brought the bacteria with them, causing another 40,000 deaths.[24] In India, the Ganges River contained the bacteria for most of the nineteenth century and became the source of most cholera pandemics, especially as ships from the British East India Company left India with infected sailors and passengers.

Cholera epidemics scared everyone, and in many people, fear generated a need to blame. A classic phenomenon in the history of medicine is *blaming the victim*. For example, Americans clung to the belief that sin caused victims to get sick with cholera. Because those who fell ill usually lived near bad water and were poor, the sick often came from groups marginalized by "proper" society. As Charles Rosenberg writes in *The Cholera Years*, "A newspaper moralist likened cholera to syphilis—scourges created to bring retribution to the transgressor of moral law."[25] For example, in Jones Valley (later the site of Birmingham), Alabama, a long creek meandered through the valley. In 1813, bars thrived by the creek, along with sex workers, poor Irish workers, and enslaved people, as well as wandering pigs, goats, horses, and chickens, many of whom used the creek for both drinking water and defecation. At the first sign of a cholera outbreak, the rich fled for cabins atop nearby mountains, where clean water, rather than virtue, saved them. Nevertheless, the rich agreed when ministers praised cholera for "cleansing the filth from our society."

Americans suffered three epidemics of cholera—in 1832, 1849, and 1866—and each time they watched as the disease started in China, India, or Russia and moved closer, sometimes to Quebec, then Montreal, and then to Brooklyn. Many Americans died in the third great cholera epidemic in America of 1866. Earlier, at Shiloh in 1862, in one of the early battles of the Civil War and, up to that time, its deadliest, 11,000 men died in two days from bullets, but a week later, cholera and typhoid killed another 11,000 in nearby Corinth.

For a long time, physicians struggled to understand the cause of cholera. For centuries, they blamed miasmas (smelly vapors). Closer to the truth, "filth theory" emerged, which hypothesized that raw sewage leaking into drinking water was not good for people, which, of course, was true. In 1854, London physician John Snow realized that cholera broke out only in the district served by the Broad Street Pump. He correctly inferred that infected water spread cholera. Nevertheless, it took years for English authorities to accept Snow's insight and translate it into good sanitation. Edwin Chadwick later convinced England to spend enormous sums to fix the problem, especially after the Great Stink of 1858.[26]

Crowd diseases came about when humans moved from the rural areas into big cities where people lived close together. This intense crowding allowed infectious diseases to easily spread in ways that didn't happen in the countryside. By 1858, great masses of people had emigrated from the countryside to London, resulting in people living with many generations in one room, even in cellars that could flood with sewage-contaminated water. Although London later became healthier and the average life-span of its citizens increased, some of the developing world today suffers similar problems—although this occurs even in advanced countries such as South Korea, as the Oscar-winning movie *Parasite* depicts.

Over centuries, people living in Asia and Europe developed a truce with these diseases, a biological homeostasis, in which those who survived passed on genes that allowed their descendants to get sick, often with flu-like illnesses, and then acquire immunity and live normal lives. As we'll see with yellow fever and malaria below, when these Europeans and Asians sailed to other continents, they brought along their diseases and unintentionally infected people there who were disease virgins.

Before the outbreak of cholera occurred in Haiti in 2010, the world had thought modern sanitation had eradicated cholera. After a devastating earthquake, the United Nations sent relief workers from Nepal to help. Unfortunately, they did not correctly construct their camps, and leakage from their latrines infiltrated local drinking water. Alas, one worker from Nepal brought *vibrio cholerae* with him, creating an epidemic of cholera on the island. Ten months after the earthquake, 665,000 Haitians became sick, and 8,183 died.[27] For nearly a decade, the UN denied responsibility, but in 2018, due to the courageous investigative reporting of Jonathan M. Katz and Renaud Piarroux, the UN finally acknowledged what had happened.[28]

Unfortunately, cholera still sickens and kills people. A highly resistant strain erupted in Zimbabwe in September 2018, infecting 10,000 and killing 69.[29]

PLAGUE

Throughout history, no word has scared people more than "plague," short for "bubonic plague" or "pneumonic plague." The bacillus *Yersinia pestis* causes *bubonic plague*, the most common and classic form. Fleas carry it, while rats and other small mammals carry infected fleas to humans. This form of plague creates inflamed swellings of the lymphatic glands in the groin and armpit, which are called *buboes*. Untreated bubonic plague kills 50 percent of its victims, although today, antibiotics treat its earliest stages. A virulent complication of untreated bubonic plague, *pneumonic plague*, destroys the lungs. When plague becomes pandemic, its pneumonic form causes the most deaths because coughing easily transmits the germ, creating chains of victims. Fearing exposure to such coughing, many fourteenth-century physicians left medicine altogether.

Like Spanish flu or cholera, victims of plague died horribly and fast. Swollen buboes soon infected their lungs and blood. Like Spanish flu, pneumonic plague could infect someone one morning and kill him the next. During the reign of Emperor Justinian in 541 CE, plague ravaged Constantinople. Because people did not know what caused plague or how to control it, it became a normal part of life in Europe, killing thousands a day. All in all, over the next two centuries and like the later Spanish flu, plague killed 50 million people.

The Black Death, the most famous pandemic in history, began in China in the mid-1300s and bedeviled European and Asian societies for the next 400 years, killing 75 to 100 million people, eventually eradicating a third of the population of Europe and a fifth of the world. During its terror, astrologers claimed that plague resulted from astrological conjunctions. More scientific types focused on swampy miasmas. Clergy said that God had sent plague to punish sinful humans. Historian Barbara Tuchman writes in her description of fourteenth-century Europe, *A Distant Mirror*, that because of the urging of clergy to atone for their sins, ordinary people hoping not to get infected in "organized groups of 200 to 300...marched from city to city, stripped to the waist, scourging themselves with leather whips tipped with iron spikes until they bled. While they cried aloud to Christ and the Virgin for pity,...the watching townspeople sobbed and groaned in sympathy."[30] In so marching, they spread fleas. When plague followed flagellants, who should be blamed? No one blamed the flagellants, but someone had to be blamed for causing this terrible situation, and some evil had to be purged to purify society. As we've seen, in many pandemics, with neither evidence nor logic, some person or group is blamed for causing the disease, a phenomenon in ethics also called *scapegoating*.

The term *scapegoating* comes from the Old Testament of the Bible, where goats were sacrificed to atone for bad things. At one time, humans were also sacrificed (hence the story of Abraham almost sacrificing his son, Isaac). In classical Mayan culture, the gods were appeased by the blood and lives of high-status humans, offered as sacrifices to ensure good crops and healthy lands. Anthropologist Mary Douglas calls these practices *purification rituals*, which reflect a typical human reaction to unexpected, lethal diseases. Such rituals exorcise impurities and restore society's health.[31] With the Black Death, Christian Europeans scape-goated Jews, who with their distinctive dress were accused of poisoning wells to spread plague. When atonement processions reached German cities, they often attacked Jewish quarters, trapping Jews inside, setting them on fire. On one day alone in 1349, marchers killed over 6,000 Jews in Mainz, Germany, just as they also killed the "Christ-killers" in Italy, Switzerland, and other European cities.[32]

In 1894, scientists discovered that *Yersinia pestis* caused plague, and within four years they had created a vaccine for it. They also taught people to control fleas to prevent plague's spread.

SMALLPOX

Breathing droplets of the smallpox virus infects people, as does touching its pustules. It scars faces and bodies of those who live; for example, we see it on the tomb-face of Pharaoh Ramses V. It afflicted the reign of Marcus Aurelius and continued into early Christianity, where Christians sometimes sacrificed them-selves in caring for victims. Europeans exploring the globe during the fifteenth century brought smallpox with them. In conquering the Indigenous peoples of North, Central, and South America, European invaders needed neither better weapons nor superior intelligence, because pandemics did their work for them. Because natives had no inherited immunity, between 1500 and 1600, smallpox killed almost 9 million of the 10 million natives on the Yucatan peninsula.[33] It took a similar toll on the Incas, facilitating Pizzaro's conquest. In North America, smallpox killed the Cherokee, Iroquois, Catawba, Omaha, and Sioux. In some cases, to hasten the demise of First Peoples, Europeans may have given infected blankets to tribes during the 1837–38 outbreak of smallpox in the Ohio Valley. One of Harvard's first presidents, Puritan pastor Increase Mather, praised God for sending smallpox to Massachusetts to kill native peoples.

In 1796, Edward Jenner created the world's first vaccine for smallpox (Chapter 6 discusses his achievement and its ethical issues). Long before Jenner's vaccine, a technique called *variolation* was used in India and Africa, where healers dis-covered the mildest cases of smallpox and scraped scabs of pus from them to deliberately infect healthy people who feared getting a deadly case. Variolation usually caused a mild infection of smallpox and immunized those who received it from deadlier disease. However, a variolated person sometimes got seriously sick and died, so the technique was not without its risks.

Increase Mather's brother, Cotton, wrote that a highly intelligent, enslaved man from Africa named Onesimus told him that he had been given a mild dose of smallpox in Africa and could not get infected again. Onesimus said the practice had existed for a century in Africa and worked. In 1716, Mather wrote to the Royal Society of Physicians in London about the practice, and five years later, during an outbreak of smallpox, he urged physicians there in his "Address to the Physicians of Boston" to try inoculation. However, racist slaveholders saw Onesimus's idea as a diabolical plot to kill them, so they resisted.[34] Evidence gradually mounted that inoculation created better survival than natural infection, so the practice slowly spread among the Colonies. During the Revolutionary War, George Washington, who had survived smallpox as a teenager, inoculated his army. Twenty years later, Jenner used cowpox instead of smallpox, creating a better form of inoculation.

In 1947, a man infected with smallpox traveled by bus from Mexico to New York City, where he became sick and checked himself into a hotel. Soon, unexplained illnesses popped up in the city's hospitals and smallpox was identified. In perhaps the most successful mass vaccination program in US history, within two weeks, hundreds of thousands of New Yorkers were vaccinated against smallpox. Dr. Israel Weinstein, the city's Health Commissioner, used the radio to passionately urge New Yorkers to get free vaccinations. Through contact tracing, authorities vaccinated citizens in a geographical ring around the first clusters— so-called *ring vaccination*. To be on the safe side, free vaccinations continued until over 2 million New Yorkers were vaccinated.[35]

In 1980, the World Health Organization triumphantly announced that all reservoirs of smallpox had been eradicated from the planet.

YELLOW FEVER

The Founding Fathers of the United States feared yellow fever more than smallpox, and with good reason. When Philadelphia was America's capital in 1793, an epidemic of it killed thousands. Before then, the disease ravaged Napoleon's troops in Jamaica and Haiti, after which Napoleon abandoned his plans to invade the Americas and sold his holdings to Jefferson in the Louisiana Purchase. In the first successful revolt of enslaved people to start a country, yellow fever killed European troops in Haiti in such great numbers that it helped enslaved people win and found their own country.

Yellow fever is caused by a virus thought to have originated in Africa in the 1600s. After a mild, flu-like illness, many Africans gained immunity to yellow fever. On the other hand, in a reversal of what happened with smallpox in the

Americas, European newcomers had no immunity to yellow fever, so it killed them in great numbers.

Infectious viruses cause varying degrees of harm in those infected. As with SARS2, most people survived the yellow fever virus, but it caused an awful death in 15 percent of its victims, with internal bleeding, such that they died by vomiting black blood (*vomito negro*), a horrible thing for relatives and health workers to witness.

Walter Reed proved that mosquitoes transmitted the virus of yellow fever to humans. In 1937, scientists created a vaccine for the disease from weakened live virus, a solution that worked well.

MALARIA

Malaria is a mosquito-borne infectious disease. It carries neither virus nor bacterium but rather a protozoan. Malaria defeated French efforts to build the Panama Canal and almost defeated American attempts to do the same. Under President Theodore Roosevelt, physician William Gorgas figured out how to eradicate mosquitoes in Panama and consequently, how to defeat malaria. Many Africans had inherited resistance to malaria as they had with yellow fever, but Europeans in Africa had not—hence its European name, "the White Man's Grave." One quirk of malaria: getting it once doesn't protect victims from getting it again.[36]

Well before the Lewis and Clark expedition (1803–06), doctors knew that quinine could cure malaria, but the best solution obviously was preventing it in the first place. The modern world controls malaria by killing mosquitoes with DDT and by using nets over beds to prevent bites.

FINAL NOTE

Why don't we know more about these past pandemics? "The final act of most pandemics is amnesia," says Howard Markel, a professor of history at the University of Michigan. "We've had plenty of warning. This kind of a crisis has been talked about for at least 20 years. But we tend to all just go back to normal afterwards."[37]

FURTHER READING

Barry, John. *The Great Influenza: The Story of the Deadliest Pandemic in History.* 2004. New York: Penguin, 2018.

Crosby, Alfred. *America's Forgotten Pandemic: The Influenza of 1918.* 1989. Cambridge: Cambridge University Press, 2004.

Diamond, Jared. *Guns, Germs and Steel: The Fates of Human Societies.* New York: Norton, 1999.

Loomis, Joshua. *Epidemics: The Impact of Germs and Their Power over Humanity.* New York: Praeger, 2018.

Porter, Katherine. *Pale Horse, Pale Rider.* 1939. New York: Library of America, 2014.

Rosenberg, Charles. *The Cholera Years.* Chicago: University of Chicago Press, 1962.

Spinney, Laura. *Pale Rider: The Spanish Flu of 1918 and How It Changed the World.* New York: Hachette, 2017.

Tuchman, Barbara. *A Distant Mirror: The Calamitous 14th Century.* 1978. New York: Random House, 2014.

CHAPTER 2
MODERN VIRAL PANDEMICS

It took scientists more than a century to learn that not all infectious diseases were caused by bacteria but that things invisible to the first microscopes caused most pandemics. These minuscule entities are called "viruses," from the ancient Greek root *vir*, which means "rod" or "path," so viruses may be seen as tiny rods seeking paths into other creatures. Today, viruses cause most pandemics, and we know that thousands of viruses surround us, replicating, mutating, and challenging our immune systems.

Occasionally, one virus crosses over from animals to humans and wreaks havoc. Consider the account of the first modern, worldwide outbreak of Ebola with Patient Zero, Charles Monet, in Richard Preston's best-seller *The Hot Zone: The Terrifying True Story of the Origins of the Ebola Virus*:

> Not long after Charles Monet died, it was established that the family of filoviruses comprised Marburg along with two types of a virus called Ebola. The Ebolas were named Ebola Zaire and Ebola Sudan. Marburg was the mildest of the three filovirus sisters.... Marburg...affects humans somewhat like nuclear radiation, damaging virtually all of the tissues in their bodies. It attacks with particular ferocity the internal organs, connective tissue, intestines, and skin.[1]

Every issue about viral pandemics has a pedigree that's crucial to understand, and those pedigrees often reveal ethical issues. We now discuss what has happened in the last hundred years with several viral epidemics and pandemics, some of which killed millions.

POLIO

Scientists had recognized the existence of polio since 1789, and during the twentieth century, periodic, localized, mysterious outbreaks of it occurred in Sweden and the northeast United States. The first outbreak in the United States occurred in 1894 in Vermont and killed 18 children and paralyzed 58.[2] An American epidemic occurred in 1916, centered around Brooklyn, New York. It killed 6,000 people and infected as many as 29,000, of whom as many as 20,000 ended up with paralysis.[3] That summer, healthy 10-year-old children swimming in lakes in New York returned home and became mysteriously ill, while something attacked their central nervous systems and destroyed their muscles, especially muscles below the waist, leaving some of them paralyzed.[4]

According to the Centers for Disease Control (CDC), "In the late 1940s, polio outbreaks in the U.S. increased in frequency and size, disabling an average of more than 35,000 people each year. Parents were frightened to let their children go outside, especially in the summer when the virus seemed to peak."[5] The worst outbreak occurred in the United States in 1952, when 60,000 were infected and more than 3,000 died.[6] Parents everywhere wondered: How could this happen? How could healthy kids almost overnight be paralyzed in the prime of their youth? What had they done to deserve this? For the remainder of their lives, some paralyzed children could only get around in wheelchairs. Some died tragically, with much attention by newspapers and radio, just as their young lives were beginning. In 1921, polio struck future president Franklin D. Roosevelt in his prime, leaving the 39-year-old crippled for life, a fact he attempted to hide from America's enemies when he became president.

By 1931, inventors had perfected the iron lung (first created in 1928), which breathed for children with paralyzed chest muscles. One person infected as a child lived inside such a machine for 50, another for 60 years.[7] Images of children in such machines burned into the minds of parents, who kept their children away from lakes and swimming pools. Eventually, scientists discovered that the poliovirus, contained in fecal material in water, caused this disease. The virus traveled from the gut to the central nervous system and later weakened muscles. In 1938, a national effort began to discover a vaccine for polio. Citizens donated to the March of Dimes, which funded the research of Jonas Salk, who successfully created a vaccine, used in the first mass vaccination program in North America. In 1955, most American children received the Salk vaccine. As we will see in Chapter 6, Salk's vaccine had some ethical mishaps, creating controversies that last until today.

As we saw with the Spanish flu, yellow fever, and smallpox, viruses affect people differently. About 75 percent of children infected with the polio virus were asymptomatic; another 20 percent had symptoms resembling the flu, and only 5 percent of children suffered badly, with their muscles not only below the waist but sometimes also below the neck becoming paralyzed. Polio broke out in small clusters in the United States again in 1958 and 1979, but scientists later eliminated these two strains. A third strain is still active in Pakistan and Afghanistan, which WHO hoped to finally conquer in 2020, but the Covid pandemic stopped its efforts, so now the virus is found in 75 percent of Pakistan's sewers.[8] Polio may also model SARS2 because most polio infections were asymptomatic or mild and its subsequent stealth transmission made it hard to stamp out.[9]

Still, from adversity, good things can emerge for some people. When the polio virus later struck film director Francis Ford Coppola at age eight, it caused him to spend a year in bed, during which he watched many films. Other famous people struck in youth by polio, and who developed their talents during their months of seclusion, include science fiction writer Arthur C. Clarke, singer Joni Mitchell, Senator Mitch McConnell, actor Donald Sutherland, Mexican artist Frida Kahlo, columnist Ellen Goodman, and actress Mia Farrow.

ASIAN FLU OF 1957 AND HONG KONG FLU OF 1968

The Asian flu pandemic of 1957 began in southeast Asia and eventually killed 2 million people. The world had not seen such a deadly flu for decades, so its emergence shocked people, as did its rapid spread in six months across the globe.

Hong Kong flu in 1968 followed the same path as the Asian flu of 1957, and although less deadly, it proved that flu could still be a mass killer. Although it may have originated in central China, this flu got its name because in July of 1968 a half million citizens of Hong Kong suddenly sickened with flu-like symptoms and swamped its hospitals. Scientists at a flu center there quickly identified the virus and alerted WHO that a dangerous new virus had appeared. The new virus quickly spread to Vietnam and Singapore, and a returning veteran from the Vietnam War brought it to Hawaii and then San Diego. It finally killed a million people worldwide, including 100,000 Americans.[10] Although the Hong Kong flu didn't sicken or kill as many as the Spanish flu, variations of this kind of virus—influenza A (H3N2)—over the last half-century have killed the most people.[11]

The first vaccine for viruses of seasonal flu came in 1936. Scientists today have identified several strains of flu, with A and B kinds and sub-kinds such as A/H1N1. The typical, yearly vaccine tries to protect against four different strains—so-called quadrivalent vaccines. Because variations of flu viruses always emerge, new vaccines must be created each year.

EBOLA

As we know, for thousands of years, pandemics from flu-like viruses have hurt humans—viruses that often originated in wild birds and bats, drifted genetically, and then spread to humans. SARS1, Middle Eastern Respiratory Syndrome (MERS), and (probably) SARS2 all originated this way. Other viruses, such as H5N1 and H7N9, came from poultry.[12]

As Richard Preston documents in *The Hot Zone*, Ebola probably moved into the larger world on New Year's Day in 1980, when reclusive Frenchman Charles Monet, who worked on the edges of a sugar plantation in western Kenya, trekked to the huge Kitum Cave on a slope of Mount Elgon, which rivals Mount Kilimanjaro.[13] The depth and width of Kitum Cave are vast, with salt crystals inside that attract elephants, so small herds often shelter inside. The cave also houses hundreds of thousands of bats. During his visit, Monet nicked his skin on a sharp crystal encrusted with guano. A week later, back at his plantation, a terrible pain emerged behind his eyeballs and his skin yellowed with brilliant red, sparkly flecks. He died a few days later in a Nairobi hospital. As he was dying, because his internal organs had dissolved, black blood spewed from his every orifice and over doctors and nurses attending him.

Had Monet simply stayed in his remote hut, the virus would have stayed there, too, but instead he flew on a crowded plane to Nairobi, passed through its airport, took a taxi to the hospital, and interacted there with hospital staff. And so the Ebola Zaire virus, its hour come around at last, slouched from its cave into the world.

Ebola Viral Disease (EVD) is deadly and quickly kills both humans and non-human primates. Officials thought it had been eradicated, but in 2014, bats infected an 18-year-old man in Guinea, where poverty and bad health systems spread it quickly to neighboring Liberia and Sierra Leone.[14] Soon it became epidemic, quickly killing 60–70 percent of those infected. Lack of protective equipment and training of medical staff, as well as traditional practices of hand-washing dead bodies before burial, spread the virus quickly across seven African countries. When an infected Liberian flew to Texas for medical care, two nurses in Dallas became infected. The Liberian died and the hospitals flew the nurses to special units at NIH and Emory. Eventually, seven other Americans became infected, including a physician who had been treating Ebola in Africa; all were quarantined, treated in the United States, and survived.

Throughout the 2014–16 EVD outbreak and under the Obama/Biden administration, the CDC modeled great leadership. During the outbreak, it trained 24,655 health-care workers in West Africa, as well as another 6,500 in the United States. It also built 24 labs to test for EVD in Guinea, Liberia, and Sierra Leone.[15] It was the CDC's finest hour.

SWINE FLU OF 1976

In 1976, an outbreak of swine flu at a military base in the United States in late winter created fears of a devastating epidemic like the Spanish flu. President Gerald Ford quickly announced a plan to vaccinate every American against it. By the end of 1976, technicians had vaccinated 40 million of 200 million Americans, nominally a great achievement. However, no epidemic developed, and the credibility of public health suffered. Still, it was wise to be safe rather than sorry.

But something else happened. A small number of vaccinated Americans then developed Guillain-Barré Syndrome, a rare auto-immune disorder and a life-long condition in which a subject's immune system overreacts and may damage peripheral nerves.[16] These events may have started the modern anti-vaxxer movement.

As we will see later in the discussion of the history of vaccines, a similar problem occurred in the Philippines when a small percentage of children died after getting a vaccine for Dengue fever. Even though the vaccine would have spared hundreds of thousands of other Philippine children from getting sick, the media followed the vaccinated children dying in hospitals so intensely that the government stopped the vaccinations.

HUMAN IMMUNODEFICIENCY VIRUS (HIV)

Like the Ebola virus, the human immunodeficiency virus (HIV) had existed for 32,000 years in wild chimpanzees, but sometime between 1900 and 1959, it infected hunters in southern Cameroon when they caught, killed, and cut up infected chimpanzees for bushmeat. When HIV-1 previously had infected Africans in this isolated area, it had spread nowhere, but by 1981, every African nation had its own international airport, so these airports and tourists became amplification systems for HIV, spreading it around the world.

By 1982, when hundreds of gay people had become mysteriously ill from a wasting disease, the CDC did not know its incubation period or its causative agent and called it GRID (Gay-Related Immune Deficiency). When babies of drug-dependent women also developed the disease, the CDC changed the name to "Acquired Immune Deficiency Syndrome" or AIDS. CDC then guessed that incubation could take years and that thousands had already been infected. At the time, no one diagnosed with AIDS had lived more than two years. In 1983, Frenchman Luc Montagnier discovered that the human immunodeficiency virus, HIV, caused AIDS.

In 1982, the CDC thought that blood could spread the agent causing AIDS and urged the screening of donated blood for hepatitis as an indirect screen for what was causing AIDS, but officials thought such screening to be too expensive. Then, by 1984, the ELISA test for antibodies to HIV had been created, which allowed HIV+ blood to be rejected. Blood banks then could have used this ELISA test to screen for HIV, but they did not. Why not? Because various groups had politicized every fact about HIV and AIDS. This politicization foreshadows the later politicization of facts about SARS2 and Covid.

AIDS and Ideology

By the end of 1981, the CDC postulated that sex among gay men in bathhouses in New York City and San Francisco probably led to the development of a bad germ, and the bathhouses acted as amplification systems for its spread. Some men there had several partners, and some of those partners traveled to other cities for sex with other partners, spreading the germ, which we now know was a virus. Cheap, easy air travel added a second amplification system.

Sharing needles and syringes to inject drugs had created yet another amplification system for this virus. Blood withdrawn from a user's vein mixes both with a drug in the syringe and with viral particles from previous users. Even community blood banks constituted amplification systems because such banks pool blood from many sources to make plasma and the clotting factor for hemophiliacs. One infected blood donor might infect dozens of recipients. Some of our modern practices also spread viruses well. As countries became more connected, with just-in-time supply chains and millions of tourists visiting remote destinations, viruses could move quickly through millions.

The 1970s had brought great changes in culture: sexual freedom spread among everyone, permissive attitudes emerged toward nonmarital sex and mind-altering drugs, and rebellion grew against authority. In medicine, psychiatrists removed homosexuality from their list of psychiatric illnesses. Unfortunately, as Randy Shilts documented in his classic *And the Band Played On: Politics, People and the AIDS Epidemic*, some evangelical Christians despised gay men.[17] Reverend Jerry Falwell blamed homosexuals for AIDS. In 1982, the secretary of Moral Majority, Greg Dixon, wrote, "If homosexuals are not stopped, they will in time infect the entire nation, and America will be destroyed—as entire civilizations have fallen in the past." In 2001, when terrorists destroyed the World Trade Center, Falwell and cable television's pastor Pat Robertson blamed gays and atheists for the event, saying it was God's punishment on heathen America.

The head of the Southern Baptist Convention similarly declared that God had created AIDS to "indicate His displeasure with the homosexual lifestyle."[18] Monsignor Edward Clark of St. John's University intoned that "if gay men would stop promiscuous sodomy, the AIDS virus would disappear from America." Conservative Patrick Buchanan piled on, "The poor homosexuals—they have declared war on nature and now nature is exacting an awful retribution." Falwell, who founded Moral Majority, a religious-political organization, advocated shutting down bathhouses. Owners of such bathhouses countered with ads extolling sexual freedom and calling Falwell a bigot. When the late, gay activist Larry

Kramer argued that shutting down bathhouses would save gay lives, gay men attacked him as a bigot like Falwell.

As mentioned, in 1984 in the midst of this controversy and with the new ELISA test available, blood banks weighed testing donated blood for HIV, but some vocal gay men resisted, arguing that their blood should not be "quarantined" and that HIV had not been proven to cause AIDS. Blood banks worried that if they screened all blood for HIV, they might lose income from rejected blood (they cannot charge for donated blood, but they charge for classifying, transferring, and storing it). In May 1984, Stanford University Hospital bravely started screening its blood for HIV. Two months later, defending a national decision *not* to screen, Health and Human Services Secretary Margaret Heckler infamously said, "I want to assure the American people that the blood supply is 100 percent safe...."[19]

It is astonishing to look back and realize that Joseph Bove, M.D., who chaired the FDA's committee overseeing the safety of the nation's blood, also chastised the "overreacting press" for causing hysteria about the safety of the blood supply.[20] Even in March 1984, when the CDC counted 73 cases of deaths from AIDS caused by transfusion of infected blood, Bove dismissed this danger: "More people are killed by bee stings." Six months later, tainted blood had caused 269 people to die.

Alas, the American government has a poor track record for being truthful during pandemics. In making their statements, Bove and Heckler either lied, were incompetent, or both. They were both political appointees by then-president Ronald Reagan, who never publicly mentioned HIV or AIDS. When politics overrules science in fighting viruses, many lives can be lost. It also seems that political appointees cannot be trusted to accurately convey medical risks to the public.

In March 1985, American blood banks began screening blood for HIV, a full year after they should have begun. Because of this lag, thousands of Americans, especially those with hemophilia, became infected with HIV. One of them, Ryan White, who had been infected at the age of 13, died at age 18 in 1990 and became a national symbol. Also in 1985, a female sex worker and intravenous drug user had tested positive for HIV. Now that she and Ryan White had the disease, AIDS seemed to be no longer just a gay disease. It had infiltrated heterosexuals and the country's blood supply.

In 1986, researchers predicted that, without treatment, almost all HIV-infected people would develop AIDS and die. That same year, a few gutsy people founded ACT UP (AIDS Coalition to Unleash Power). Its demonstrations forced the FDA, and the head of the National Institute of Allergy and Infectious Diseases—a certain Dr. Anthony Fauci—to shorten by two years its process for approving new drugs. By 1987, AZT (zidovudine) became the first anti-HIV drug. ACT UP also forced Big Pharma to allow Indian companies to sell generic versions of anti-HIV drugs to developing countries.

As of 2020, about 40,000 new cases of HIV were being diagnosed each year in the United States and about half lived in the rural South; about 18,000 were young Black men.[21] There is still no vaccine for HIV. When no treatment existed for HIV, contact tracing for those possibly HIV-infected became fruitless. Many people asked, "What's the point? Why do I want to know I have an infection that will soon kill me in a horrible way?" When treatment came, things changed. In South Africa, when clinics provided HAART (Highly Active Antiretroviral Therapy) to those infected, many of those contacted decided to get tested.

Cuba and AIDS

Of relevance to the quarantine in Wuhan, in 1986 the authoritarian government of Fidel Castro in Cuba sent all HIV-infected Cubans to a camp, the Sanitorium, at the edge of its island, where they had to live for the rest of their lives. Perhaps from guilt at such an extreme measure, Cuba made this camp nice—far nicer than the conditions in which most Cubans lived. Some Cubans, called "frikis," deliberately infected themselves with HIV to get in. Why? Castro associated rock music with the United States. Because of this, his police arrested rock musicians, aka "frikis" (weirdos, freaks), and forced them to work like slaves in cane fields. Friki leader Papo la Bala decided that life inside the Sanitorium would be better, so he deliberately injected himself with HIV+ blood. When HIV+, la Bala went to the Sanitorium. Afterwards, 200 more frikis followed. Being HIV+ became part of the identity of the frikis. Inside the Sanitorium, they made music and lived as they liked. On rare occasions outside, their HIV+ status kept police away.[22]

After eight years, Cuba relaxed this policy and required only eight weeks of education for first-time, misbehaving infected Cubans; repeat offenders went to the Sanitorium for life. After AZT and protease inhibitors became available, making HIV a chronic condition and not a terminal diagnosis, quarantine was no longer necessary and in 2016 Cuba closed the Sanitorium.

If good jobs require proof of immunity from Covid, and if poor people cannot get easily vaccinated, we might see "Covid frikis" arise, where poor workers deliberately infect themselves, recover, and then get certified to work.

SARS1

In the spring of 2003, a coronavirus named Severe Acute Respiratory Syndrome (SARS1) originated in China. Scientists already knew about coronaviruses, which form a spectrum and include the viruses causing common colds. Many non-human animals, such as bats and small mammals, experience coronaviruses and carry them. We now know that the SARS1 virus originated in Asian palm civets, leapt to cave-dwelling horseshoe bats in China's southwest province of Yunnan, and then jumped to humans.[23] SARS1 left China on airplanes and went to Hong Kong and Canada. In February, a woman infected 257 people in Toronto; infections from an orthopedic ward there infected another 361. Panic ensued, and thousands of Toronto's citizens voluntarily quarantined in their homes. For a few months, those staying inside feared Asians, whom they blamed for the virus.

Singapore, with an authoritarian government, identified 8,000 citizens who had been exposed to the virus and isolated them against their will, but it did compensate them for lost income from missing work (Canada did not compensate workers missing work, resulting in widespread noncompliance). SARS1 also taught lessons to Taiwan and South Korea—lessons burned into their memories about quickly containing initial outbreaks through testing, contact tracing, and quarantine that helped them later control SARS2.

It is useful to compare the clinical course of SARS1 and SARS2.[24] Although most who caught SARS1 survived, many afterwards had long-term problems, including shortness of breath, chronic lung disease, and kidney problems. Even three years after the outbreak in Toronto, many survivors experienced musculoskeletal pain and fatigue, similar to lasting problems with the Epstein-Barr virus. This seems to imply that some of those infected with SARS2 will experience long-term problems, a topic discussed in the next chapter.

Altogether SARS1 infected less than 9,000 people and killed about a thousand. Why it disappeared is little understood.

SWINE FLU OF 2009

On April 15, 2009, a novel influenza virus (H1N1pdm09) emerged in California and soon spread quickly across the world, causing the first global pandemic in four decades. It scared epidemiologists because, like the Spanish flu, it was a novel H1N1 virus that spread rapidly. The new virus contained elements from birds, humans, and pigs, a combination that made a new hybrid of a Eurasian pig-flu virus, hence the name "swine flu."

Six days later, the CDC began working on a vaccine, and four more days later, the WHO declared a "public health emergency of international concern." On April 24, the CDC uploaded the genetic sequence of the new virus to an international public database for scientists to use to find vaccines and treatments; four days later, CDC released a test to detect the virus. By June 25, a million Americans had been infected and by August, four strains had appeared that resisted treatment by standard anti-viral drugs.[25] Unlike seasonal flus that killed mainly people over 65, swine flu killed like Spanish flu: primarily young adults and the middle-aged under 65, as well as some children.

In July, clinical trials of a new vaccine began, and by September, the CDC had approved four vaccines. By December, 100 million doses were available, and in January, President Barack Obama declared January 10–16 to be "National Influenza Vaccination Week," hoping to get all Americans to take the H1N1 flu vaccine,[26] which the president took in front of reporters a week later. By its end,

31

swine flu had killed about 12,000 Americans and infected about 60 million, but it was nothing like the Spanish flu and not much worse than normal flus. The quick creation and rollout of a vaccine helped a lot. Hindsight is always perfect, and critics accused the WHO of overreacting in declaring an emergency, some even claiming its declaration was designed to help sell vaccines—a claim discredited by independent investigators.[27]

Several European countries used a different vaccine, called Pandemrix, that contained an oil-in-water emulsion adjuvant called AS03 (adjuvants are substances mixed with vaccines to increase the body's uptake and integration of the vaccine). Especially in Finland, those getting the vaccine had an increased risk of unexpectedly developing narcolepsy, caused by disturbances in the brain's ability to regulate sleep–wake cycles. Pandemrix has not been used against any flu since 2009.[28]

MIDDLE EASTERN RESPIRATORY SYNDROME (MERS)

September 2012 saw an outbreak of a coronavirus in Saudi Arabia called "Middle Eastern Respiratory Syndrome" (MERS-CoV), which caused severe breathing problems and killed 35 percent of those infected.[29] At first linked to hospitals in Saudi Arabia, over the next eight years, authorities documented about 2,500 cases. It also spread to other countries on the Arabian Peninsula and to South Korea.

At present, there is neither a treatment nor a vaccine for MERS, but it did not become pandemic because, like leprosy, it requires sustained, close contact to spread. Outside of hospitals, its spread is rare, because it may only be linked to close contact with camels. Although it has not vanished, most humans outside the Arabian Peninsula have little risk of getting it.

ZIKA

In 2015, many babies were born in Brazil with microcephaly—unusually small heads. An old virus, Zika, had mutated and become dangerous, causing Zika Virus Disease (ZVD), whose symptoms included not only microcephaly but also other brain/eye defects and development disorders.[30] A common mosquito, *Aedes aegypti*, spread the mutated virus. A year later, the Zika virus had spread to 60 countries. Through 2016 and 2017, Brazil had nearly 3,000 babies born with ZVD.[31] In addition, the CDC predicted that nearly 1 million Puerto Ricans had been infected by Zika in 2016 and that eventually 80 percent of those would be infected. Before Hurricane Maria hit in September 2017, officials had been tracking 4,000 babies born of mothers infected with Zika, but after the hurricane devasted the island, tracking stopped.[32]

Because the Zika virus was likely transmitted in blood, in 2016 the FDA required blood banks to screen for it. After not screening blood initially for HIV, the FDA had learned its lesson. Although this decision added $8 to the cost of a unit of donated blood, it saved some babies from microcephaly.

For unknown reasons, Zika cases plunged dramatically in 2018 in both the United States and elsewhere in the Americas. Only one American became infected with Zika from a mosquito.[33] Why Zika disappeared is unknown, much like the disappearance of Spanish flu, SARS1, and other diseases.

OTHER VIRAL DISEASES AFFECTING HUMANS

Many other viruses cause diseases in humans. The diseases include forms of herpes (simplex, types 1 and 2), human papillomavirus (causing venereal warts and cancer), several kinds of hepatitis (B, C, E, and D), Lassa fever virus, rubella virus, Varicella-zoster virus, Epstein-Barr virus (causing chronic fatigue syndrome), Norwalk virus, rhinovirus, dengue fever virus, West Nile virus, measles, the mumps virus, and dozens of other viruses causing lesser-known diseases in humans.

Finally, we should be skeptical when someone says, "It's just the flu." Between 2012 and 2019, seasonal flus each year typically killed 22,000 to 61,000 Americans—no small number.[34] In fact, wearing masks and sanitizing hands to combat Covid greatly reduced the number of flu cases in 2020, proving the efficacy of such measures.

FURTHER READING

Loomis, Joshua. *Epidemics: The Impact of Germs and Their Power over Humanity.* New York: Praeger, 2018.

Preston, Richard. *The Hot Zone: The Terrifying True Story of the Origins of the Ebola Virus.* 1994. New York: Anchor Books, 1995.

Shilts, Randy. *And the Band Played On: People, Politics and the AIDS Epidemic.* New York: St. Martin's Press, 1997.

CHAPTER 3

THE MEDICAL NATURE OF SARS2

The End of October, a novel published in 2020 by Lawrence Wright, could not have arrived at a scarier time.[1] Revealing years of careful research, the book describes a lethal virus that breaks out in Indonesia, evades attempts to contain it by the Centers for Disease Control (CDC) and World Health Organization (WHO), travels to the annual Hajj in Medina where it is amplified thousands of times, and then races around the globe, destroying societies and creating a "Bladerunner" future. Although a pessimistic view of our ability to contain such viruses, it did assume a non-politicized CDC and WHO, which now seems too optimistic.

This chapter discusses the medical nature of the SARS2 virus and the clinical course of Covid, the disease caused by SARS2, as well as long-term problems of those once infected with the virus.

DISPUTED ORIGINS OF SARS2

Long before SARS2 appeared, experts had predicted such an outbreak to be inevitable. To understand the SARS2 eruption and to prepare for future ones, we must understand where such viruses come from and how they infect humans. Over 300,000 viruses infect all mammals, including bats and birds, but to date, just 220 have infected humans.[2] However, given how viruses replicate and mutate, new lethal viruses will always emerge.

Since the emergence of the SARS2 in late 2019, many have queried how it started in Wuhan and then spread around the globe. Several major theories have emerged. The first, supported by the Chinese government, holds that the virus jumped from bats to humans in an open wet market in Wuhan that sold and butchered live animals. Such markets often lack good sanitation, and the close proximity of live animals to humans makes them ideal for viruses jumping between species, becoming hybrids, and taking on traits from each species that give the hybrids new properties (for more on this, see below). Such new properties may include the ability to infect humans, as is seen with SARS2.

After China demolished the wet market and all evidence of what had been sold there, conspiracy theories blamed China for a cover-up. In fairness, demolishing such a market to eradicate any remaining virus is the first thing good public health should do. A problem with the first theory is that there were no bats for sale at the Wuhan market. Some scientists proposed that another animal, such as a pangolin, was a carrier for the virus and brought it to the market, but it has not been proven that pangolins were for sale there either. Moreover, most bats in China live 1,000 miles south of Wuhan, which makes their sale in Wuhan unlikely. Finally, it was winter in Wuhan, when bats hibernate.

Another theory involves the fact that much research is done on bat coronaviruses at the Wuhan Institute of Virology by its famous scientist, Shi Zhengli, aka "the Bat Lady." Some say this institute, when dealing with hazardous diseases, had a history of violations regarding proper disposal of research animals and proper use of protective equipment. According to this line of thinking, a worker in this lab acquired a virus from a bat, created a hybrid, and then carried it outside the lab.[3] Indeed, then-secretary of state Mike Pompeo, a Congressman who had been elevated to the position by President Trump and who had little experience with foreign affairs, claimed that the virus came from a Chinese lab. Without citing any evidence, Senator Tom Cotton claimed on Fox News that China had engineered the virus as a weapon. Such scapegoating involved the Trump administration's attempt to blame China for the pandemic.

A third theory holds that the coronavirus was a human-made biological weapon that mistakenly got released. This theory has been largely discredited, in part because the virus wasn't that lethal, so it would have been a poor weapon. But the Web erupted with other weird theories, such as one claiming that Chinese citizens got the virus from eating a delicacy called "bat soup." When China finally let WHO researchers into Wuhan in 2021 to investigate and disclosed 174 (allegedly) asymptomatic cases that started as early as November 2019 and with no connection to the Wuhan market, it did not help rebut conspiracy theories that China then refused to give researchers raw data that could have confirmed where and how the first cases occurred.[4]

Occam's Razor is a principle of explanation in science that holds that simple theories are the best. Put differently, if one must choose between a simple theory and a complex one that makes many assumptions, the simplest one is likely the more accurate. In this case, in the southeast Chinese cities of Kunming or Guangzhou, millions of Chinese live near bat caves, and bats from such caves emerge most nights to eat insects, during which time bats urinate and defecate. Some people there trap bats for sale in markets that sell live animals. We already knew that each year a million people are infected in this area by viruses from bats.[5] In the case of SARS2, what probably happened is that when trapping, transporting, and selling bats, someone became infected with a mutant coronavirus that spreads easily among humans. Perhaps only that person's family became infected and perhaps they lived outside the city on an isolated farm, so the virus didn't spread. At some point, someone infected with SARS2 traveled to Wuhan's crowded wet market, as well as to other places in China, where it probably circulated for weeks before the official outbreak. When enough people became suddenly ill in Wuhan in December 2019, doctors suddenly took notice. Although the exact way in which this virus emerged may be important in the blame game, the more important point is that, given wet markets, overpopulation, and the number of people living in close proximity to bats, it was inevitable that such a virus would emerge.

Antigenic Drift and SARS2

Germs come in three broad classes: protozoa, bacteria, and viruses.[6] Viruses, by far the smallest of these organisms, replicate with frequent errors and thus mutate frequently. The reservoir for most viruses resides in non-human animals, especially bats and birds, and close contact of such animals with humans allows animal viruses to intersect with human viruses to create new, hybrid viruses, some of which become dangerous to humans.

Viruses vary greatly, and a single virus may change over time. After a few years, some viruses weaken or disappear (viruses for Spanish flu, Zika, and common colds), while others never go away (the HIV virus). This changeability of viruses makes their future course difficult to predict. A new virus might seem dangerous, authorities might quickly create a vaccine for it, but then, after millions have been vaccinated, it might weaken to not be a threat.

Crucially, most flu viruses that affect humans come about through an important process called *antigenic drift*. When they replicate, viruses are unstable and prone to errors. As microbiologist and pandemic historian Joshua Loomis explains,

> Every time influenza viruses invade new cells and begin to replicate, the new genomes that are made contain small mutations. This is important because it increases the chances that a brand-new and deadly strain will emerge and ravage the population. This process by which influenza viruses mutate gradually... [is] antigenic drift. It is... why we must be inoculated with the flu vaccine annually: the flu strain present during one flu season may mutate enough the following year... that our immune system no longer... recognizes it.[7]

37

The capacity of a virus to damage its host is called its *virulence*, and its capacity to spread is called its R_0 *value* (pronounced "R-naught"). An R_0 of 1 means that a virus affecting one person typically infects one other person, while a R_0 of 3 means a virus infecting one person typically infects three other people. The R_0 of most colds is around 1, but of SARS2, it's over 2. Some of the variants of SARS2 have both a higher R_0 value and are more virulent.

Variants of SARS2

Variants of the original coronavirus in Wuhan mutated, as is common with viral replication and antigenic drift, producing more transmissible strains than the original.[8] By November 2020, a variant emerged called "Cluster 5" that infected mink farms in Denmark and eventually infected 200 people, causing the government to kill 17 million minks, destroying a $760-million business as an attempt to prevent the spread of this hybrid virus to more Danes.[9] Minks also become infected in the Netherlands and Spain, where authorities destroyed them, and in the American states of Utah, Wisconsin, Michigan, and Oregon.[10]

By December 2020, scientists had identified a thousand variants of SARS2.[11] By April 2021, three dangerous variants of SARS2 had erupted, one in Britain (B.1.1.7, or simply B117), one in South Africa (B.1.351 or B1351), and one from Brazil (P.1 or P1).[12] Other variants known to infect people had also been detected in California, New York, and Oregon. Originally predicted to be slow to produce variants dangerous to humans, SARS2 evolved faster than expected and quickly produced several variants. Controlling such variants may be the most important long-term problem caused by SARS2 (a topic revisited in the final chapter).

By mid-December 2020, B117 had infected a thousand British people, was about 50 percent more infectious than SARS2, and was, according to Britain's Health Secretary, "out of control."[13] By April 10, 2021, the United States had 20,915 cases of B117, which dominated new cases, the majority of which erupted in Michigan and Florida.[14] At the same time, with some countries having only 6 percent of their citizens vaccinated, B117 spread quickly in Europe, leading to major lockdowns in Paris and Germany, where it caused the majority of new cases. In London, the UK variant comprised 96 percent of viral samples at Britain's three major labs.[15] The United Kingdom had the world's best system for genomic sequencing of viral samples, giving it advance warning of dangerous new variants. Because North America lacked similar testing, it once again flew blind, barely able to track new variants.

Lack of knowledge of rising cases of variants may hobble future efforts to return to normalcy. In Britain and continental Europe, a high plateau of cases of the original strain masked the rise of B117, especially when vaccinations started to curb the original strain. Only Britain's extensive testing prevented it from being ambushed by B117, and even then, it took three months of hard lockdowns and aggressive vaccinations to check it. Lacking such testing, B117 silently grew in Poland, the Czech Republic, Germany, and France, allowing huge numbers of new cases to erupt. In the United States, speedy vaccinations and reduced testing may similarly mask the rise of variants, so its 75,000+ new daily cases in April 2021 may similarly enable the rise of variants. In December 2020, the United States tested only a few hundred samples a week for variants. New CDC Director Rochelle Wallensky pushed that to 9,000 per week in late spring, and the Biden administration pledged $200 million to test 25,000 samples a week for variants.[16]

All these variants seemed to have higher R_0 values than the original Wuhan strain. The UK variant also had greater virulence. Worse, the South African strain, accounting for 5 percent of cases in France in early 2021, may have reinfected some people previously sickened by the original Wuhan strain.[17] Some of the variants contain a mutation called E484K (or "Eek"), which allows the variant virus to evade immune responses induced by the Pfizer and Moderna vaccines, and even more so, the AstraZeneca, Johnson & Johnson, and Novavax vaccines.[18] Because of the danger from these variants, several European countries banned flights from Britain. Japan, with its aging population, closed its border and banned foreigners at its Summer Olympics in 2021, an event that had already been postponed from the previous summer.[19]

The Brazilian variant (P1) looked both deadlier and more virulent—especially to young people—than the original strain, devastating Brazil, by April 15 killing over 350,000 people, more than in India or Mexico and second only to the United States. At the same time, the United States discovered 500 cases of P1, and Canada detected 877 cases, centered on the ski resort of Whistler, making British Columbia the biggest cluster of cases outside of Brazil.[20] The South African variant (B1351) seemed to evade Oxford's AstraZeneca vaccine, such that South Africa switched to the Johnson & Johnson vaccine.[21] By April 2021, it had taken hold in France, Belgium, Luxembourg, Sweden, and Norway.[22]

The increased R_0 values of SARS2 variants illustrate several things: first, antigenic drift, which constantly creates new variants; second, evolution, because in the struggle of survival among viruses, more infectious viruses reproduce themselves more successfully and triumph over less successful ones. Lastly, even as much as the world suffered pandemic fatigue, outbreaks of new, more virulent strains might best be thought of as separate epidemics, each of which needed a strong response. To help the public understand variants, in 2021 the CDC created three classes of such variants: those of (1) high consequence, (2) concern (B117, B1351, and two variants originating in California: B1427 and B1429), and (3) interest (P1, and two variants originating in New York: B1526 and B1525).[23]

These SARS2 variants also illustrate how virulence can increase. With the Spanish flu of 1918, it took eight to nine months for a more lethal strain to emerge in Europe and to travel back to North America (where the most damage occurred). Similarly, with SARS2, it took about eight to nine months between the first case in Britain and the emergence of the new UK strain. To evolve in this way, a new variant needs both large reservoirs of the original virus in a population and large numbers of people susceptible to new infections, which was true in 2021 with SARS2 in the United States, South Africa, Brazil, Russia, and Europe.

THE CLINICAL COURSE OF COVID-19

Clinical Course and Medical Treatment of Covid

Early on, people who resented the lockdowns caused by attempts to stop the spread of SARS2 claimed it "was just another kind of flu" or "no worse than the flu." They claimed that, given how many died each year from a seasonal flu, SARS2 would not kill any more. This is false. SARS2 and the disease it causes, Covid, are more lethal than most seasonal flus. Moreover, unlike ordinary flu, significant numbers of Covid patients experience symptoms many months after their initial infections. And, of course, flu is not just a common cold. Every year, it kills as many as 60,000 Americans, especially seniors and those with compromised immune systems, which is why reasonable people take flu vaccines each year.

Once SARS2 enters humans, it hijacks their cells, as if to say, "Don't do your usual job. Your job is now to help me multiply and help me make virus."[24] Typically entering through the mouth and sinus passages, SARS2 "crawls progressively down the bronchial tubes" to enter the lungs, where it inflames mucous membranes, often damaging lung sacs and making it more difficult for the lungs to deliver oxygen to circulating blood.[25] From the lungs, the virus may go on to enter the gastrointestinal (GI) tract, other organs, and perhaps even the brain.

Roughly 20 percent of people infected with SARS2 need medical treatment, and about 5 percent of those require hospitalization. The classic list of symptoms of initial infection with SARS2 includes loss of sense of taste and smell, fever, chills, and anything that involves the lungs, such as a dry cough or shortness of breath. As physicians learned more, the list of initial symptoms expanded to include muscle aches, headaches, GI upset, diarrhea, muscular pains, swollen testes, and skin rashes. In rare cases, unusual rashes appear on fingers and toes, dubbed "Covid toes."[26] At some point the virus may enter the brain and central nervous system (hence, loss of taste and smell). Long-term studies of patients reveal that viruses may linger in the brains and central nervous systems of some patients for months, maybe years. Such patients are called "long haulers."

As noted above, about 80 percent of infected people have mild or no symptoms. The other 20 percent experience serious flu-like illness. In the United States, the SARS2 virus has killed about 2 percent of those infected, especially the elderly, those overweight, and those with underlying medical problems. It easily infects smokers and vapers.[27] It kills men over 50 much more than women over 50, for unknown reasons, and more often, men of color.[28] However, the 2-percent mortality rate of SARS2 might be exaggerated. At one time, CDC estimated that for every known infection of SARS2, another seven asymptomatic cases might exist in people never tested but who would have antibodies. If that were so, the true mortality rate of SARS2 would be less than one-quarter of 1 percent.

Why then were American hospitals overwhelmed with patients sick with Covid? Not so much because SARS2 is so lethal but because it is so infectious: two to three times more infectious than seasonal flu viruses. If hundreds of millions get a new infection they otherwise wouldn't have, and then even if it kills only one-quarter of 1 percent of them, that's still a lot of deaths (over 577,000 in the United States). The 5 percent who are hospitalized in intensive care units (ICUs) take up enormous resources of equipment, staff, and money, often staying for months. They are hospitalized partly because they are mostly older and suffer from other serious medical problems. Those over 65 with such problems comprise 15 percent of the American population but 85 percent of Covid deaths.

Care for Covid patients in hospitals is expensive. Because ICU beds are limited, as they filled up in states such as New York, physicians faced ethical dilemmas about whom to admit or discharge, with the most heart-wrenching question being whether they should evict a patient who is likely to fail and die in the ICU in favor of a new patient who is likely to recover (Chapter 5 discusses these issues). Patients sometimes had mild symptoms the first week and then suddenly got very sick the second. In those infected, lack of oxygen could be critical and often went undetected, such that by the time they entered the emergency room, oxygen levels in their blood were dangerously low. (Inexpensive pulse oximeters, which fit like a finger-puzzle toy on a finger, easily detect such levels.) The first cases in China and the United States received mostly supportive care. Early in the pandemic, physicians put very sick patients on ventilators, sometimes splitting one scarce ventilator among two patients, but today they try to prevent this, using ventilators only as a last resort. Because some patients on ventilators stay in the hospital for months, the toll on their organs and minds is great, such that full recovery may take months or even years, leaving some with "brain fog."[29]

Monoclonal antibodies, such as those made by Regeneron and given to then-president Trump in October 2020, block viral replication and, if given early, seem to help. Today, physicians intervene aggressively to avoid ventilators, using steroids, supplemental oxygen, monoclonal antibodies, and the anti-viral drug Remdesivir, as well as *proning* (turning patients frequently so they can breathe more easily).[30]

Because the coronavirus is so infectious, hospital staff treating patients must wear personal protective equipment (PPE) resembling suits worn by astronauts. This means that family members cannot touch or visit sick relatives. Sad scenes on television show relatives waving to patients outside nursing homes, seeing each other only through glass windows. As one doctor put it, "You die of coronavirus all alone."[31]

Immunological Storms

Recall that the Spanish flu killed mainly younger people aged 20 to 40. One explanation traditionally has been that previous generations had often been exposed to bad seasonal flus and developed immunity to them, but then two decades passed without serious flus and produced "flu virgins" with little immunity who were at-risk when the really pernicious virus came in 1918.[32] However, in recent times a better theory has evolved that emphasizes the role of *cytokine storms* in the immune system, caused by both the virus of the Spanish flu and SARS2. The immune system normally functions as a balanced system where, if too weak, infections, cancers, and other diseases occur, and where, if too active, autoimmunological damage occurs as the system acts against itself rather than against foreign material. The basic idea of cytokine storms is that for some people, for reasons not completely understood, the immune system that normally does a good job warding off germs goes too far and vastly overreacts.[33] This overreaction in some causes much more damage than the invading germs themselves.

Cytokines are immune-signaling molecules that activate immune cells and help them align against pathogens. They have long been studied in rheumatology for their role in autoimmune disorders.[34] When they overreact and when too many are released quickly, a cytokine storm occurs, a bad thing because the overreaction itself can damage cells and tissue, causing cytokine storm syndrome and even death.[35] Because they did not create cytokine storms, individuals infected in 1918 with Spanish flu with weak immune systems paradoxically fared better than those with strong systems storms. Clinicians treating very sick Covid patients now often suppress immune responses by giving steroids to avoid cytokine storms.

Immune systems vary in people. Over a hundred genetic varieties exist of immune deficiencies. The most common congenital immune deficiency involves low levels of antibodies.[36] About 2 percent of people with SARS2 fare poorly, and they may have "enhanced IL-1-beta responses" or "perforin pathway mutations," which may cause cytokine storm syndrome. About 40 percent of African Americans inherit genetic polymorphisms associated with enhanced IL-1 production, compared to only 6 percent of Caucasians. This could help explain why African Americans, when infected with SARS2, die more often.[37]

How Deadly Is Covid?

Epidemiologists who count Covid deaths worry that we first notice a pandemic when very sick patients arrive in hospitals, but that doesn't tell us how many patients were infected and never got sick. Many people get the flu virus every year, but most easily survive. Overall, until they randomly sample the general population, epidemiologists don't know how deaths from Germ X relate to general infections for Germ X. This problem may explain why early estimates for deaths from SARS2 infection were too high, such as Ferguson et al.'s estimate of 2.1 million US deaths and 250,000 deaths in Great Britain.[38] Ferguson et al.'s report did not distinguish between deaths where the virus was the proximate cause in people with other serious medical problems and deaths solely caused by the virus, nor did it emphasize that 70 percent of those hospitalized would be over 80 and that nearly 10 percent of deaths would be in those over 80, that is, people with a high likelihood of dying from other causes during the next year.

Six months into the pandemic, several studies put the rate of death of those infected at between 0.5 and 1 percent, meaning that for every 1,000 infections, between 5 and 10 people on average would die.[39] Covid, then, is worse than seasonal flu but not as bad as the Spanish flu of 1918 or Ebola. The Spanish flu killed half a million Americans, equivalent to killing 1.6 million Americans today. However, these facts belie the seriousness of Covid. As Eric Toner, an ER physician and senior scholar at Johns Hopkins Center for Health Security, explains, "It's not just what the infection-fatality rate is. It's also how contagious the disease is, and Covid is very contagious. It's the combination of the fatality rate and the infectiousness that makes this such a dangerous disease."[40] Put differently, if SARS2 eventually infects all the people on the globe, that's 7 billion people. Even 0.5 percent of that figure is a big number: 35 million deaths.[41]

It is common to compare deaths for typical years pre-Covid with those during Covid, noting that deaths are far higher after Covid started. Statisticians call this the *problem of excess deaths*. From February 1, 2020, to February 6, 2021, excess deaths in the United States compared to the previous year were over half a million (536,566).[42] Across the globe, excess deaths were over 3 million.[43] But how many of these deaths were caused by the coronavirus? The problem is that lockdowns also cause deaths. Lockdowns cause unemployment, depression, abuse of relatives and children, excess drinking, drunk driving, deaths from opioid overdoses, and avoidance of hospitals. All of these factors could cause rates of death unrelated to infection by SARS2 but nevertheless related to the pandemic. Lax or late reporting of Covid deaths also caused problems. When sick patients overwhelmed hospitals, taking time to create accurate statistics was often a luxury.

A final point is worth noting, too. As deaths surpassed 577,000 in the United States and hospitals suffered, skilled staff became scarce. During the first year of the pandemic, *Kaiser Health News* tracked 3,470 Covid deaths among American health-care workers: those on the front lines treating those who had been infected, a feat for which it won prizes in journalism.[44]

Cardiopulmonary Resuscitation (CPR) and Covid Patients

A flashpoint in clinical ethics consultations has concerned whether and how to do cardiopulmonary resuscitation (CPR) on Covid patients. Just how infectious are SARS2 aerosols created by CPR on a Covid patient? Doing CPR on Covid patients became a big ethical issue when medical workers were faced with performing chest compressions with inadequate PPE.

One of the unexpected requests to the Medical Ethics department at Cornell Weill Medical Center in New York City during its surge of cases in March 2020 was whether the team had to do CPR on an infected Covid patient with dementia who had little chance of returning to normal life.[45] Unless a patient had a signed DNR order, New York State required CPR. An additional ethical issue arose when PPE was scarce or unavailable, especially face shields. At least one scholar concluded that medical staff were not obligated to perform CPR on Covid patients without good PPE.[46] In general, once you understand that chest compressions create aerosols in a patient's room, CPR becomes a dangerous procedure, one in which the team seeks a definite benefit from taking high risks.

CPR amidst Covid surges presents a unique challenge, as crisis standards clash with existing norms. Ideally, medical teams should determine in advance when CPR should be administered, especially when staff lack good PPE. Daniel Kramer of Harvard Medical School and colleagues recommend that rather than trying to save every life, the crisis standards of care take on a utilitarian nature by maximizing lives—both present and future—saved under severely limited resources. They advocate ethical principles of fairness, transparency, respect for the patient, and honoring decisions of surrogates while balancing risks to essential workers, especially from inadequate PPE.[47]

With terminal Covid patients, planning about CPR ideally needs to occur in several parts: discussing plans of care and DNR status with families and being honest about limited resources. With severe medical problems or advanced age, forgoing CPR should be presented as an ethical option because keeping hospital staff safe in this way may be necessary. Finally, only when essential workers have donned PPE for intubation should resuscitations begin.

Infected Children
Although most children experience SARS2 with mild or few symptoms, some suffer bad reactions. For some, a cytokine storm may occur called *multi-system inflammatory syndrome*. At first, doctors thought such children had the rare Kawasaki's Syndrome, but they later decided that multi-system inflammatory syndrome was the correct diagnosis. As of March 21, 2021, over 3,185 children in 48 states and Washington, D.C., had the condition, and 36 had died of it.[48] Tragically, its mean age of onset in children was eight years old. Strangely, and what is worrisome to parents, many children did not even know they had been infected with SARS2 and then, six to eight weeks later, became so ill that they were rushed to the hospital. In more than a thousand cases in children with this syndrome, a large study found that 75 percent experienced no symptoms at initial infection.[49]

As with elderly Covid patients, a large percentage (63 percent) of affected children were African American or Latinx, and 60 percent were male, suggesting a genetic predisposition. Many were also overweight, but we need to be careful mentioning this fact because it can be code for "so they are to blame for getting sick and not controlling their weight." Still, any connection between Covid and obesity should be explored, particularly with respect to children suffering from multi-system inflammatory syndrome.

TRANSMISSION AND IMMUNITY

Transmission of SARS2

As former president Donald Trump told journalist Bob Woodward late one February 2020 night in a recorded phone call, SARS2 spreads more easily than seasonal flu. And as scientist Anthony Fauci has said many times, "This is a highly infectious virus." So how exactly does this virus spread? We know that the coronavirus easily spreads through airborne transmission and not easily on surfaces.

Because its definition has been controversial, it is important to define "airborne transmission." At first, the WHO's definition included only the transmission of large, airborne droplets communicated at close range, for example in a sneeze. But a pioneering scientist at Virginia Tech, Linsey Marr, whose career has been spent studying aerosols, warned the WHO in June 2020 (with 213 fellow scientists) that tiny aerosols could infect people as easily as droplets. She was correct. That fact matters for prevention. Tiny aerosols travel farther and stay airborne much longer than droplets. As a result, in poorly ventilated rooms, physical distances of six feet will not prevent the virus's spread when an infected person coughs.[50]

Take someone—call her Anne—who has been exposed to an infected person—call him Shawn. Anne sat near Shawn at a bar, with neither wearing face masks. How likely is it that Anne will become infected? This likelihood depends on three variables: (1) the viral load in Shawn at the time, (2) for how long and how closely Anne sat next to Shawn, and (3) and whether his airborne particles went directly into Anne's lungs. For example, exposure in a crowded, noisy bar where Shawn shouts close to Anne's face for more than 15 minutes will more likely infect Anne than if she were merely walking in a park six feet away from him. Of course, extended bodily contact from kissing, massaging, or sexual intercourse between Anne and Shawn would dramatically increase the likelihood of transmission of SARS2.

Wearing masks dramatically reduces the spread, as researcher Monica Gandhi, of the University of California at San Francisco Medical Center, has argued. In a famous study by the CDC of a hair salon in Springfield, Missouri, two infected stylists wearing masks over 10 days did not infect any of their 139 mask-wearing customers.[51] Dr. Gandhi also emphasized a poorly understood fact: wearing a mask also protects the person wearing it: "So, it really is based on the fact that we've known for many years now—probably a hundred—that the more virus you get into your system, the more likely you are to get sick."[52]

SARS2 can be detected on surfaces for some time, but it rapidly degrades there, especially in open air and with sunlight. In April 2021, the CDC said the chance of getting the virus from a surface was less than 1 in 10,000.[53]

Closed-loop, indoor air circulation systems in restaurants and on airplanes might transmit aerosolized viral particles, but again, much depends on the volume of virus in the air. Airplanes and restaurants that draw in lots of fresh air dramatically reduce the concentration of the virus indoors, and those that filter air through HEPA filters reduce concentrations even more. Thermo Fisher Scientific has made an air sampler that not only successfully detects SARS2 particles in the air but also captures them.[54] Because circulation systems on commercial airplanes suck in great amounts of fresh air, the risk of transmission of aerosolized viral particles should be low on such planes.

One study in 2020 frightened medical staff because it revealed that the virus could spread in hospital air much farther and more easily than previously believed.[55] Florida researchers collected live virus from aerosols seven to 16 feet away from Covid patients. This study carried ominous implications for anyone working indoors in cold weather locked inside sealed buildings with no fresh air, upping pressure there to equip the HVAC systems with HEPA filters.[56] As the weather turned cold and people stayed indoors closer together, transmission by aerosols caused new surges of infection. Lower humidity and colder temperatures made the coronavirus more virulent.[57] Some research suggests that when heated air dries mucus membranes and because viruses last longer in colder, drier conditions, people working inside in cold temperatures are more easily infected, creating an ethical issue of how best to protect workers in meat-packing plants, who tend also to be poor and people of color.

Community Spread

At the start of 2020, SARS2 seemed to be transmitted only by people with symptoms and fever. If SARS2 were an infectious disease like Hansen's disease (leprosy), only long, prolonged, direct exposure around infected people would infect others. But SARS2 is very transmissible between people. With some infectious diseases, it is relatively easy for scientists today to track the spread of infections. This occurs with *point-of-origin outbreaks*, such as when fecal matter containing the cholera bacterium contaminates a well in a rural area. Authorities can track everyone who used the well, close down the well, and shut down the outbreak. Alas, most viral spread comes from a different pattern. When new viral diseases emerge, it is not always easy to understand how they spread and by whom. When they seem to be spreading from people without symptoms to others without symptoms, *community spread* occurs, a technical phrase meaning "it is spreading in the community and we can't easily track who will infect others and who will get infected."

At the beginning of the outbreak in Wuhan, Chinese authorities denied community spread, but alert physicians warned that it was occurring. Early on, they suspected that SARS2 was highly infectious. One brave physician, Li Wenliang, an ophthalmologist, treated many sick Covid patients and became the first physician in Wuhan to die from the virus. By June 2020, the virus had killed five more Wuhan physicians.

Super-Spreaders

Super-spreaders are individuals with a high viral load who interact with many people in business and personal life as they speak, cough, yell, sneeze, or sing, spreading lots of virus around them. A super-spreader appears to have sparked the outbreak of the Hong Kong SARS1 virus in 1968. Certain people appear to be viral super-spreaders. Typical super-spreaders have no symptoms when they infect others, and even when symptoms appear, they exhibit only mild symptoms, making them invisible and identifiable only in retrospect.

Super-spreader events figure prominently in community spread of SARS2. In February 2020, 175 personnel of Biogen met at a Boston hotel, and one of them had SARS2. Those attendees spread the virus to an estimated 300,000 people across the United States.[58] Another infected person at Mardi Gras in New Orleans in February 2020 fueled 50,000 infections in the South.[59] A rally in Sturgis, South Dakota, attracted 490,000 defiant motorcycle riders, many not wearing masks and crowding into bars, probably infecting millions.[60]

Although children do not typically get sick from the virus, they may spread it to adults.[61] At a summer camp in Georgia in June 2020, about 600 children and dozens of staffers tested negative in the week before attending the overnight camp, but some must have become infected after testing because the virus entered the camp, and some got sick. The 344 people who developed symptoms were tested again, and 260 (76 percent) were positive, including 231 children and 29 adults.[62] CDC concluded, "These findings demonstrate that SARS-CoV-2 spread efficiently in a youth-centric overnight setting, resulting in high attack rates among persons in all age groups, despite efforts by camp officials to implement most recommended strategies to prevent transmission. Asymptomatic infection was common...."[63]

Post-Infection Immunity and Reinfection

Evidence is slowly accumulating about whether those who have recovered from infection have immunity against new infections or reinfections, and if so, how long it lasts. It seems certain that the older one is, the shorter one's immunity because the immune system of seniors is not as good as those who are young. As will be discussed in Chapter 10, the length of immunity is important for countries and entities that issue immunity certificates, also called status certificates.

Whether and how immunity may occur after infection with SARS2 is not completely known. In some people, antibodies that resist the virus appear soon after infection and last at least six months. In seniors, similar antibodies generally last much less time, maybe only a few months. Whether such antibodies protect against reinfection is not completely known. Also, because this kind of virus is constantly creating variations through antigenic drift, it is not known whether recovery from the original SARS2 virus will confer immunity against variants of it. Whether vaccinations give the same length of immunity as infections is under study, but it appears that Pfizer and Moderna vaccinations may do as well or better than actual infections, giving at least six months of protection and maybe more. Both companies planned to monitor original test-subjects for two years.[64] Both vaccines seem also to prevent both symptomatic and asymptomatic infections.[65]

Reinfection does seem to occur. Hong Kong researchers documented a man who became infected in China in March, recovered, repeatedly tested negative for the virus with a PCR (polymerase chain reaction) test, but four and a half months later became reinfected in Europe. Previously, researchers thought that such cases were dormant viruses re-emerging, but in this case, "researchers at the University of Hong Kong sequenced the virus from the patient's two infections and found they didn't match, indicating the second infection differed from the first."[66] Professional cyclist Ferando Gaviria contracted Covid in February racing in Saudi Arabia, tested negative by PCR test for eight months, and then tested positive by PCR test in Italy in October. Over 275 cases of reinfection are thought "probable" worldwide, with another 2,500 cases "suspected."[67]

More troubling are some cases where previously healthy people have been infected and hospitalized several times over the months following initial hospitalization. In one case, a 54-year-old Michigan man was hospitalized seven times. As medical reporter Pam Belluck summarized, "Data on rehospitalizations of coronavirus patients are incomplete, but early studies suggest that in the United States alone, tens of thousands or even hundreds of thousands could ultimately relapse (or get infected by a new variant) and return to the hospital."[68] A CDC study of over 100,000 Covid patients hospitalized between March and July 2020 in the United States found that 1 in 11 had to be re-hospitalized over the two months following discharge.[69] The Brazilian variant (P1) also reinfected Brazilians who previously had a bout of Covid, but it was unclear which strain they first had.

Anthony Fauci says that cases of reinfection occur but that "it's unlikely that this is replication-competent virus," meaning that the virus is not replicating itself but also not entirely disappearing. It's also true that "other people recover and then get clinically ill, and they come back, and it looks like it's a positive test. Is it residual? Is it reinfection or is it exacerbation? The answer is, we don't know."[70]

Herd Immunity

Herd immunity is an important concept and may refer to having about 70–90 percent of a population immune to an infection or illness, either through vaccination or through prior exposure. The underlying idea is that not every member of the herd needs to be immune in order to protect the whole herd. Vaccinating children against measles is a good example, where about 90 percent of children must be vaccinated to protect most children, even the unvaccinated ones.

When the reproductive number (R_0 value) of a virus is above 1, the infectivity of the virus often follows a bell curve. As the virus keeps finding new people to infect, and they in turn find others to infect, the number of cases soars.

With viruses such as Ebola, two people can infect four people, who infect eight people, who in turn infect 16 people, and because the increase is exponential, soon hundreds of thousands are infected. By the end of a pandemic, the number of cases creates a bell-shaped curve, with a slow spread at the beginning, and without efforts to stop it, an exponential increase, and finally, as the population gains immunity, a taper.

Therefore, two populations curb viral spread and flatten the bell curve: those previously exposed and those vaccinated. For example, if everyone in a population is susceptible, the initial curve of the virus keeps soaring, but if 40 percent of the population has had the virus and if another 40 percent has been vaccinated, then only 20 percent of the population remains to be possibly infected. This means that the virus, when it encounters 10 people, will likely infect only two of them, and thus the rate of new infections starts to rapidly drop.

Like other key terms about pandemics, "herd immunity" is not a clear, unambiguous phrase. For example, what is the "herd" immune from? Is it immune from death? Hospitalization? Is it immune from transmitting the virus to others, what immunologists call *sterilizing immunity*, the complete absence of the virus? Is it about the virus becoming undetectable, even in long-haulers? However it is defined, herd immunity differs for different germs. As noted above, protecting children by herd immunity from measles requires 90 percent of children to be vaccinated. Herd immunity from seasonal flus is far lower, around 70 percent. What will it take for there to be herd immunity from SARS2? Part of the answer depends on how it's defined, and the other part depends on the passage of time.

Long Covid: Patients with Continuing Symptoms

Although SARS2 is new and not completely understood, some patients, after their first infection wanes, experience symptoms afterwards for many months or even a year.[71] At first, physicians dismissed their complaints as due to anxiety or as over-reactions, so these patients formed groups online to share stories. They call themselves *long-haulers*, like truckers who work long hours hauling goods around the country with little appreciation from society.[72] One such long-hauler, Chelsea Alionar, on March 9, 2020, had a terrible headache and soon could not smell or taste. Three months later, she still had numb fingers and toes and forgot familiar words.[73] A Facebook group for long-haulers, Survivors Corps, in early 2021 had over 150,000 members.[74] In a study of 1,733 patients, six months after discharge from a Wuhan hospital, 75 percent had at least one of these symptoms: insomnia, fatigue, depression, diminished lung function, or anxiety.[75] Some had their hair fall out.

History tells us that this is not unexpected. One-quarter of people in Hong Kong who had SARS1 in 2003 ended up with myalgic encephalomyelitis (ME), a chronic condition characterized by loss of memory and attention (aka "brain fog") and extreme fatigue after mild exertion.[76] Anthony Fauci says that "Long Covid," as long-haulers' condition is termed, may be best understood as a version of ME.[77]

The immune system here may be confused about clearing SARS2, constantly creating immunological storms that cause victims to suffer. New clusters of ME are linked to outbreaks of several other viral infections, so we can predict Long Covid in substantial numbers of those infected with SARS2. This gives the lie to television stations' apparent compulsion to emphasize good news when reporting about the pandemic, especially the tendency to follow latest statistics about infections and deaths with the good news of how many have "recovered." If one-quarter of those infected with SARS2 get Long Covid, instead of classifying them as "recovered," we should acknowledge that we are facing an enormous group of people who present a long-term health-care crisis. Significant numbers of adolescents and children experience Long Covid. Some of them had few symptoms at initial infection but afterwards experienced fatigue and problems of memory or concentration, often for months. In spring 2021, the Kennedy Krieger Institute at Johns Hopkins University established a special clinic to help such patients, and at about the same time, Long Covid received the scientific name "post-acute sequelae of SARS-CoV-2 infection."

That many patients upon initial infection lose their sense of taste and smell means the virus has invaded the part of their brain and central nervous system responsible for these senses. Neurologists think the virus invades neural cells and may alter the brain. It also enters the central nervous system, causing inflammation and then causing strokes or Alzheimer's disease.[78] When viruses invade the brain, they can stay there a long time, as is the case with the Epstein-Barr virus.[79] It is therefore understandable that SARS2 in the brain has long-lasting effects. According to Igor Koralnik, Chief of Neuro-infectious Diseases at Northwestern Medicine in Chicago, "thousands" of patients who survived Covid experience Covid brain fog, a loose diagnosis that includes loss of memory, confusion over simple tasks, difficulty finding the right words, and dizziness.[80] As one nurse said after recovering physically, "I feel like I have dementia." A study of nearly 4,000 members of Survivors Corps found that over half report difficulty concentrating or focusing. In March 2021, at Mount Sinai's center in New York City for Long Covid patients, some had been experiencing symptoms for over a year and required six to 12 months of therapy.

A 2020 study of MRIs of the hearts of SARS2 patients showed some with cardiac abnormalities. German researchers compared scans of the hearts of a control group of patients of the same age and gender with a group of 100 Covid patients, months after their infection, and discovered that the Covid patients had such abnormalities.[81] Worries about getting Covid and damaging their bodies caused some professional and college athletes to opt out of the 2020 season.

Understanding one possible fact about the coronavirus may explain an important ethical issue involving long-haulers. It is likely that fragments of the coronavirus reside in internal, reservoir organs of infected patients. These organs, deep inside the body, are immune-privileged and lack immune-mediated cells.[82] Nevertheless, parts of the viral RNA of SARS2 may make the patient infectious and exhibit symptoms. What's also important is that long-haulers may still be infectious. Because of the location of the viral fragments, even a deep nasal swab may miss them, so long-haulers can test negative while retaining the virus. Many months after infection, many long-haulers report problems sleeping well. Preliminary results indicate that melatonin blocks transmission of the virus or its development into Covid.[83] This may also be indicated by how melatonin regulates sleep in the brain. Doctors also report that a few patients experienced psychosis following infection, usually temporary but in some cases requiring treatment with anti-psychotic medication.[84]

CDC recommends that home isolation can end after three days with no fever, and after respiratory symptoms improve. Unfortunately for long-haulers, fever and troubled breathing can come and go, so when do they stop self-isolation? Equally important, when are they no longer infectious? When are immunity certificates good for them? As we will discuss in later chapters, what is the implication of long-haulers for challenge studies for vaccines, that is, volunteers who agreed to be infected to study vaccines (see Chapter 6)? If a vaccine doesn't work and volunteers agreed to be infected with SARS2 and end up being long-haulers, is there any compensation from society? Do long-haulers pressure the ethical permissibility of the original challenge studies?

Canadian psychiatrist Jeremy Devine argues the contrarian view that "Long Covid is largely an invention of vocal activist groups" and lacks rigorous scientific evaluation.[85] Although it may be true that many victims of Long Covid claimed this status without actually being tested for SARS2 and that hundreds of symptoms have been claimed to be due to Long Covid, most physicians believe that Long Covid is real and that the $1 billion allocated by the NIH to study it is appropriate.[86]

In sum, long-haulers first present special problems for physicians and relatives, who should not dismiss the symptoms of such patients as fictitious or due to anxiety. Whether and when they are infectious should be studied, and we need better tests for viral particles deep inside them. Second, long-haulers raise numerous ethical problems about status certificates, challenge studies for experimental vaccines, and effective periods of isolation or quarantine.

FURTHER READING

Centers for Disease Control (CDC). "COVID-19." https://www.cdc.gov/coronavirus/2019-ncov/index.html.

Cron, Randy Q., and Edward M. Behrens, eds. *Cytokine Storm Syndrome*. Cham, Switzerland: Springer, 2019.

Kucharski, Adam. *The Rules of Contagion: Why Things Spread—And Why They Stop*. New York: Basic Books, 2020.

Lostroh, Phoebe. *Molecular and Cellular Biology of Viruses*. Boca Raton, FL: CRC Press, 2019.

Sontag, Susan. *Illness as Metaphor*. New York: Farrar, Straus and Giroux, 1978.

CHAPTER 4

POLICIES FOR CONTAINMENT

Do a just society's national values strive only to prevent deaths in fragile citizens, or could other national values exist, such as economic prosperity, preventing teenage suicide, or preventing military attacks? Bioethics has always been linked both with medicine and with medical personnel and, as such, is oriented to the values of medicine. In pandemics, the goal of such values is to save the most lives, prevent the most illness, and protect medical personnel. Yet outside medicine, other values exist, which may be difficult to articulate. Inside medicine, unexpected deaths during pandemics are unacceptable, but parts of the general public may see things differently: for example, in one poll in 2020 when 176,000 Americans had died of Covid, 57 percent of Republicans thought that if the economy could be kept open, that number of deaths was acceptable.[1]

QUARANTINE AS A PREVENTIVE ALLOCATION STRATEGY

"Quarantine" is a scary word, one especially so for democracies that value liberty. The United States used its first quarantine facility, its *Lazaretto* for maritime immigrants, not on Ellis Island, but between 1797 and 1799 outside Philadelphia to contain yellow fever. "Lazaretto" stems from the parable of the beggar Lazarus and Jesus. Often islands in harbors, such as Manoel Island in Malta, Robben

Island in Cape Town, or San Quentin in San Francisco, Lazarets could also be old ships at permanent anchor. Until certified as safe, enslaved Africans imported to Georgia typically quarantined at Tybee Island. In 1912 in Washington state, just across the river from Astoria, the US Government built a lazaretto, which is now a museum.

Quarantine operates on many levels. China locked citizens of Wuhan inside its borders and banned all travel. It also stranded its citizens abroad and forbade foreigners from entering. Japan and Australia did the same. This is how real quarantine works. In the movie *Dr. Zhivago*, General Strelnikov is ruthless in his fight against the old Russian aristocracy. He seems cruel but successfully furthers his goals. So the generals of quarantine must be ruthless: loved ones must be stranded abroad, new hires must be rescinded, no one can be allowed to leave or re-enter the country—not even for funerals, marriage, to treat cancer, or for organ transplants. Any exception, no matter how worthy, allows germs to enter.

Exceptions quickly lead down a slippery slope. Compassionate leaders could easily allow infected relatives to enter a quarantined country, destroying the basic premise of quarantine. Critics of US immigration policy hate chain immigration—the way in which one member of a family can become a permanent resident, then later bring in a spouse or children, then grandparents and so on, a chain that seems to have no end, especially because there can be blended families or extended families. But with quarantine, once you allow an exception, you permit a germ to enter, setting off a chain with much deadlier consequences.

The Diamond Princess Cruise Ship

After officials in Hong Kong notified Japan that a passenger on the ship had disembarked in Hong Kong on January 25, 2020, and tested positive for SARS2, the cruise ship Diamond Princess approached the Japanese port of Yokohama on February 3, with more sick passengers on board, so Japan quarantined the ship's 3,711 passengers and crew for 14 days. Two days after its arrival, 10 of its passengers tested positive. The Japanese government hoped that the virus would not spread on board and that only symptomatic passengers needed to be isolated. Because of how air circulated on the ship and because of asymptomatic transmission (although this was unknown at the time), within three weeks, the virus infected 700 people on board. On February 21 (day 18 of quarantine), Japan allowed passengers ostensibly free of infection to leave, leaving 1,300 on board.

A study in the *Journal of Travel Medicine* found that on "the cruise ship, conditions clearly amplified an already highly transmissible disease" and that evacuating the ship sooner could have stopped the spread, resulting in fewer cases.[2] The CDC concluded that the quarantine of the ship had contributed to 700 infections and nine deaths (Johns Hopkins estimated 13 deaths). In the case of this quarantine, not allowing passengers to leave saved infections of local Japanese but spread infection onboard. Even 17 days after all passengers had left the ship and after the ship had been disinfected, investigators still found RNA of the coronavirus in the cabins, creating problems for the cruise industry about how to safely re-open.[3] Japan eventually paid 94 percent of the costs of medical treatment for foreigners on board who became infected.[4]

FOUR MODELS OF FIGHTING PANDEMICS

1. The Total Approach

The Total Model (or Total, for short) to fighting pandemics aims to totally elimi-nate the virus from a society by all necessary means. All other values—per-sonal liberties, economic health, even medical emergencies—suddenly become abandoned as all resources, including military and local law enforcement, are marshaled to eliminate a dangerous new germ. China employed Total aggres-sively to control the spread of the virus: using quarantine, shutting down schools, businesses, and resorts, and using contact tracing. Very aggressive, Total is utili-tarian, emphasizing containing lethal germs quickly inside a locked-down area, accepting the loss to the disease of some inside for the greater good, and banning all travel to or from the locked-down zone to protect the rest of the nation.

Total employs the *cordon sanitaire*, made famous in historical quarantines, where no exceptions can be made about people entering or leaving, no matter who they are or what their relation is to those inside. Next, any outbreak must be met swiftly with quarantine, contact tracing, and public support. Also, everyone must be tested as often as possible to gauge the spread of the germ. Last, a robust system of public health must be in place to implement the above measures. Total inflicts pain swiftly, to the economy, to personal liberties, and to families, with the goal of avoiding the greater pain later of massive infections, massive hospi-talizations, numerous deaths, and economic misery.

On January 23, 2020, with the imminent start of the Lunar New Year when a billion of its citizens planned to travel, China quarantined Wuhan and imple-mented Total, shutting down shops, canceling all public events, and using its military to prevent anyone from leaving the city. By February 4, Wuhan had 8,351 cases. To handle them, China furiously built two temporary hospitals, with a thousand beds each, on cleared land inside Wuhan, a process televised to the world, which prayed that the new virus could be contained there. Although China's internal political system discouraged any broadcasting of bad news about the country, and thus delayed medical news about the outbreak, once national authorities realized that a dangerous virus had erupted, they responded with unprecedented aggressiveness. Soldiers sealed huge apartment complexes, allow-ing no one to leave and delivering food and medical supplies to those locked inside. Houses containing infected, but less seriously sick, citizens were locked from the outside. Policed roadblocks prevented anyone from leaving the city by car. Trains stopped running and planes stopped flying.

Less than two weeks after Wuhan's first 8,351 cases, officials ordered everyone in Wuhan to stay inside their homes. All businesses were shuttered; all K–12 schools closed; Wuhan University sent students home and locked remaining foreign students inside; no one could even exercise or walk in public parks. The city became a ghost town. Only police and soldiers could travel outside, along with couriers, who delivered everything. Fearing shortages, people hoarded food, medical supplies, and toiletries. Both heavily controlled by Chinese authorities, television and the Internet provided the only contacts with the outside world. Doctors and nurses, often pressed into service outside their specialties, could not go home to their families but lived at government expense in hotels and dorms. One nurse left for work on February 3 and didn't return home until June 7.[5] Doctors and nurses in other cities, in return for dangerous service in Wuhan, were offered admission to elite schools for their children.

Local committee officials controlled neighborhoods and blocks in China's cities such as Wuhan, and they enforced the rules in ways unimaginable to Americans and others outside China. Grandmothers and aunts surveyed their local streets like little czarinas, spying on everyone, enforcing every rule. On a larger scale, China used facial recognition technology to monitor its citizens, as well as regulating WeChat, a phone app almost universally used in China. Soon after the lockdown of Wuhan, China also banned travel inside its country. By March 24, the virus had spread to 300 cities in China, infecting 80,000 people. But China soon had the virus under control. It moved aggressively against the smallest outbreaks. It eventually tested each of Wuhan's 8 million citizens for the virus. By October 2020, China had re-opened businesses and movie theaters in Wuhan, as well as travel to and from the city. When the United States topped 10 million infections, India 9 million, and Brazil 6 million, China by this time had fewer than 100,000.[6] When the United States had 240,000 deaths, China had (officially) fewer than 5,000.

By using Total, China saved millions from getting sick and hundreds of thousands from dying. Had it adopted Focused Protection or Intermittent Lockdowns, both described below, tens of millions could have died in its huge, crowded cities. On the other hand, citizens in affected areas had very little freedom and were virtual prisoners in their own homes.

2. Focused Protection

Focused Protection takes a softer approach to controlling the virus, avoiding quarantine and shutdowns of schools and small businesses, opting instead for targeted interventions.[7] It is associated with two economists who called it the "Great Barrington Project," arguing that the pandemic could be contained without the drastic methods of Total.[8] Focused Protection rejects the assumption that a just society first and only prevents deaths from Covid of medically fragile people. It argues that economic shutdowns can create greater harms. Focused

Protection ensures the safety of the people who get otherwise hurt or killed in Total.

Consider 10 of those harms: (1) Lockdowns caused millions to lose their jobs, especially in restaurants, bars, amusement parks, resorts, travel, tourism, and casinos. (2) Lost jobs cost some people their homes or got them evicted. (3) Feed America has estimated that one in three families in the United States suffered from lack of food. (4) Deaths from drug overdoses and alcoholism increased from 69,000 in March 2020 to 81,000 in March 2021. (5) Domestic violence increased. Staying home all day, with alcohol and drugs being added to existing tensions in a family, led to more violence erupting against partners, children, seniors, even pets. (6) Civil unrest increased as protests flared over lockdowns, loss of jobs, and wearing masks. (7) Children were damaged, as their early learning and socialization were interrupted. College students missed opportunities for research, internships, study abroad, and athletic competition. (8) People with disabilities were hurt. People with special needs require extra, expensive contact, which withers during lockdowns. (9) Suicide and despair increased: people need interaction with others, so without a social life, they decline and lose interest in life. In Japan alone, nearly 7,000 women, mostly single, committed suicide in 2020, often from loss of jobs and enforced isolation. In India, due to Covid and new policies, 30,000 farmers committed suicide (described below). (10) Many small businesses failed, and in North America such businesses account for most jobs, so some economists predict it may take a decade to recover.

If the first theme of Focused Protection is that the costs of Total Lockdowns are too high, its second theme is that societies can defeat germs without shutting down everything. Thus, Focused Protection uses what is sometimes called the "Swiss Cheese Defense," which imagines many overlapping slices of Swiss cheese, each slice with holes in it where viruses can pass through, but taken together it is a solid block of prevention. Ian McKay, an Australian virologist, built on the work of others in industrial safety and started the Swiss Cheese Respiratory Pandemic Defense, which requires many layers of protection and cooperation to stop viral spread.[9] For example, McKay says masks must not only be worn by everyone, but also be worn correctly, frequently washed, have multiple layers of cloth woven tightly, and be disposed of correctly. Another slice of cheese is physical distancing, which McKay says is the most effective preventive. Countries that stopped SARS2 used many aspects of the Swiss Cheese Approach: limiting travel into and across their borders, providing safe places for infected people to quarantine and paying salaries while they did so, circulating fresh air in buildings, and creating clear, transparent, evidence-based messages.

Rather than complete shutdowns, Focused Protection advocates reduced capacity at gyms, bars, restaurants, and stores to 20 percent, which allowed many to limp along but also stopped the spread of the virus in large gatherings.[10] Such capacity limits work best in areas where the incidence of the virus is low. Florida focused on protecting vulnerable elderly in nursing homes, but otherwise it enforced few measures to limit the virus. A year into the pandemic, both it and New York state had about 2 million cases and nearly 40,000 Covid deaths, but Florida's economy and tourism were booming. New York may not have done enough to protect its citizens in nursing homes and may have under-reported deaths there for several months, an omission that became a scandal for Governor Andrew Cuomo.

A variation of Focused Protection is to target closings by zip codes and businesses rather than having mass closures: for example, closing a Chuck E. Cheese where families tend to stay for hours but allowing a McDonald's with less density and quick turnover to stay open, or allowing restaurants to stay open in a county with an incidence of the virus under 2 percent but closing them in counties with incidence over 10 percent.[11]

The problem with Focused Protection is that it may assume widespread compliance with the behaviors needed in each slice. It will not work in countries where citizens are divided over the dangers of the virus, where the behavior of some makes new holes in the cheese. Focused Protection may also work well if vaccinations are administered quickly, as has been occurring in Israel, Great Britain, and the United States. With no vaccinations, or very slow rollouts of vaccinations, more strenuous measures may be needed to control the spread of the virus, as happened with the lockdown in Paris in March 2021. On the other hand, others argue that governments that imposed severe lockdowns lacked a coherent way to calculate the costs and benefits of such lockdowns, compared with the looser policies of Focused Protection.[12]

3. The Swedish Approach

Sweden took a different approach to the virus, not closing schools and not mandating wearing masks. Seeing itself as a relatively healthy, young country, it decided that a softer approach might work better for its citizens. As such, it instituted very few layers of the "Swiss Cheese Defense" and let the virus run its course.

Citizens around the world in lockdowns saw pictures of Swedes in bathing suits crowded together on wharfs and beaches—an eerie, open-air experiment. Because Sweden didn't shut down its economy, North American businessmen pointed to Sweden as the ideal. Although Sweden's prime minister never claimed it as a goal, Sweden's chief public health officer, Anders Tegnell, implied that its goal was to quickly achieve herd immunity among Swedes through controlled exposure. In Sweden, the public health officer has great authority.

Critics said that Sweden's approach would sacrifice fragile senior citizens through achieving herd immunity and that it would take at least a year to achieve that. But Tegnell argued that critics had misconstrued Sweden's plan, imputing bad motives to them. Rather than sacrificing their grandparents to the virus, Tegnell argued, he was saving Swedes from other harms, such as suicide, increased addiction, domestic violence, and poverty. In discussing Sweden's approach, Thomas Frieden, the former CDC director under Barack Obama, said that if the United States followed Sweden, the cost of achieving herd immunity by letting the virus run its course would be "the deaths of one million Americans."[13]

Sweden had some justification for its approach. With its comprehensive medical system giving free medical care to all citizens, Swedes did not fear losing medical coverage through loss of jobs or high co-payments for being sick. As one Scandinavian said, "You're not as concerned about catching the virus, because you know that, if you do, the state is paying for your health care."[14] However, Sweden was widely criticized by officials in public health and medicine, who focused on the value most dear to them—saving lives. In the midst of a deadly, worldwide pandemic, these health-oriented officials did not value non-medical values as much, for example, the loss of intensive education for children or suicides of teenagers in lockdowns.

Six months into the pandemic, only 10 percent of Swedes had immunity to the virus, and neighboring Norway, Finland, and Denmark had banned Swedes from entering their countries. At this time, Sweden's death rate exceeded that of the United States—564 per million citizens in Sweden versus 444 in the United States[15]—and was nearly five times that of the combined rate of its four nearby Nordic countries.[16] In 2021, Sweden ended its gamble, banning gatherings of more than eight people, as its hospitals struggled to handle all the sick Swedes and as its death toll passed 8,000 in one month, the highest toll in a month for Sweden since the Spanish flu of 1918.[17]

4. Intermittent Lockdowns

Intermittent lockdowns are not really a well-thought-out approach to a pandemic, but a mixed bag, reflecting deep ambivalence about the correct steps and how far to take them. Because politicians during pandemics face tension between satisfying businesspeople and controlling infections, countries may lurch back and forth between these poles. The great dangers are waiting too long to lock down and then re-opening too soon.

In this approach, we will distinguish between soft and hard lockdowns. The United States had soft, temporary lockdowns without fines or imprisonment for violating rules about masks, distancing or gatherings, as well as haphazard and spotty curfews. Soft lockdowns imposed loose requirements for quarantine, often voluntary or at the citizen's expense and without anyone checking to see if those contacted really quarantined. Hard lockdowns, say on a college campus, designated a dormitory or hotel where those exposed were required to stay and where they were monitored, sometimes with electronic leashes. Hard lockdowns in Ontario, Canada, had strict curfews, often of long duration. Hard lockdowns controlled the virus much more effectively but hurt businesses more.

SUCCESSES AND FAILURES AROUND THE WORLD

Africa's Dilemma

Coronavirus kills those older than 60 at a much higher rate than those under 20, whom it rarely harms.[18] The virus killed so many in Italy partly because 23 percent of Italians had reached age 65.[19] Those living in the wealthiest countries generally live the longest—countries in North America, Europe, and the wealthy countries of Asia. In Japan, for example, the median age is 48.[20] But the average age in Africa in 2020 is 19.7 years, and what is even more amazing is that those under age 15 make up 40 percent of the hundreds of millions of people on that continent. Only 6 percent of Africans live past 60.[21] Lack of birth control and abortion, the need for young children to help run farms, and the desire to produce enough children that some survive to take care of parents in old age—all of these factors contribute to Africa's tsunami of young.

Consider the Republic of Niger, a huge, landlocked mass intersected by the Niger River and bordered by seven countries. On the UN Human Development Index (informally, the "Happiness and Misery Index"), Niger ranks 187th out of 188—one of the world's poorest countries. Niger also boasts the youngest median age in the world, age 15—over half its people are under age 20, and 75 percent are under 30. On October 25, 2020, Niger had only 1,200 SARS2 infections and 69 Covid deaths.[22] Niger contains an estimated 25 million people, but only around 1.5 million are over 60. By adopting Total or several strong lockdowns, Niger could destroy the lives of 20 million young people, perhaps giving its age 60+ citizens their statistical few more years.

Total, therefore, would not work in Niger. Would even intermittent lockdowns work in the country, with its open borders and a weak government? Probably Niger's best hope is to use the Swiss Cheese Defense and possibly sequester its elderly in safe places. The fact that Niger, along with other developing countries in Africa and South America, contains so many young people alters what plan might work best for them, making Total and Intermittent Lockdown unattractive and Focused Protection more so. In Niger, Focused Protection could be called the "Business/Youth" model, for the two groups it seeks to protect. In addition, for reasons not yet understood, the death rate from Covid in Africa is nothing like that of North America and Europe. Despite minimal systems of public health and hospitals, Nigeria's (not Niger's) death rate is less than one-hundredth of the US rate.[23] Except for South Africa, similarly low death rates hold for most of sub-Saharan Africa. Given such facts, why should countries such as Niger and Nigeria not adopt the Swedish approach?

Because of the crowded conditions of the townships outside Cape Town, the virus hit South Africa hard at first, growing in five months from one case to half a million. As a result, its government, like India's, suddenly imposed one of the most severe lockdowns in the world, certainly harsh for a democratic country, even suppressing the sale of alcohol. But its extreme ("Level 5") lockdowns in the townships did not work well.[24] Instead, they imposed severe hardships on the poor. Perhaps the mitigation measures of Focused Protection would have been just as effective.

If we interpret utilitarianism as dictating that right acts produce the greatest number of life years for the greatest number of people (see Chapter 5), then it is not only permissible for Niger to adopt Focused Protection; it is morally required to do so. Similarly, in the townships of Cape Town, in the sprawling cities of India and Indonesia, Focused Protection might be the most beneficial approach, despite what that means for medically fragile elders.

Intermittent Lockdowns: Italy and Germany

Europe, Great Britain, Canada, and the United States employed Intermittent Lockdowns with varying degrees of success. As such, if Total is the extreme of restrictive infection control and the Swedish approach is the least restrictive, then Intermittent Lockdowns lie in between.

Italy first experienced SARS2 when two Chinese tourists and an Italian brought the virus from China to northern Italy. By mid-February 2020, Italy had 16 cases and soon quarantined the provinces surrounding Milan, suspending all travel in or out of the region and declaring a state of emergency. But it was too late, as the virus overwhelmed Milan's hospitals, killing so many that the army evacuated corpses in convoys to mass graves—images carried on cable television around the world, and which should have warned North America about its future.

When the virus spread outside Milan, in March then–prime minister Giuseppe Conte closed all businesses except grocery stores, pharmacies, and hospitals. Soon a quarter million Italians had been infected and 35,000 had died. Citizens even needed forms to prove to police they needed to go outside their homes. Through these draconian measures, by August, when the United States was experiencing 100,000 new cases a day, northern Italy had none.[25] Italy had to maintain constant vigilance against the virus. In so doing, it banned tourists from the United States and the United Kingdom and extended Prime Minister Conte's emergency powers. In doing so, it angered many, including Italian philosophers such as Giorgio Agamben, who argued that a return to fascism might occur.

After months of long lockdowns, citizens in Italy, as well as in Spain and the United Kingdom, resumed normal activities in the summer of 2020, attending family gatherings, weddings, and parties. However, even though the spread of the virus had slowed, it had not ceased. It was like fighting a forest fire to get it under control, then abandoning efforts to fight it by opening up, so the fire grew again. When colder months forced people inside, cases skyrocketed after Halloween. In the United Kingdom, Prime Minister Boris Johnson then imposed a month-long hard lockdown, hoping to save the British economy's lucrative Christmas season; Prime Minister Conte ordered hard lockdowns in Italy for the same reason, resulting in the loss of many jobs and widespread anger. France and Ireland imposed similar lockdowns. Germany imposed a more targeted lockdown in the fall, more along the lines of Focused Protection, but it didn't work well, so before the week of Christmas, Chancellor Angela Merkel announced a strict lockdown and urged employers to offer employees a holiday until January 2.[26]

Resistance mounted to these new lockdowns. Italians were sick of them. In the United States, even Anthony Fauci questioned whether long, hard lockdowns were necessary, urging everyone to simply mask and socially distance. In the United Kingdom, Manchester's mayor, Andy Burnham, even urged citizens to defy lockdowns. In December, Prime Minister Conte imposed severe restrictions on travel on Italians for the high-travel days surrounding Christmas and New Year's Day, limiting them to travel within their region. He also imposed a national curfew of 10 p.m. and limited how bars and restaurants could open in hot zones.

Germany combined aspects of Focused Protection and Intermittent Lockdowns in containing the virus under the leadership of its chancellor, Angela Merkel. Whereas the United States narcissistically wanted its own test and bungled it, Germany developed a diagnostic test quickly, in January 2020, which the WHO subsequently distributed worldwide. Chancellor Merkel and her medical advisors quickly established three principles: (1) the template for making the test would be made available to the 200 public and private German labs, (2) the test would be free for everyone, and (3) other testing would be sidelined for rapid turnaround of SARS2 tests.[27] If their results were negative, Germans could do as they pleased. If they were positive, they had to self-isolate. Like many other European countries, Germany restricted travel and mandated social distancing, letting only essential businesses remain open.

Thanks to a well-funded system of public health that began there under the vision of Germany's first chancellor, Otto von Bismarck, in the nineteenth century, Germany was in a good position to fight the virus. First, public medical insurance covered about 90 percent of Germans. Its *Kurzarbeit* system paid factories not to lay off workers but instead to retain them on short hours.[28] Because of Chancellor Merkel's leadership during the previous decades, Germany had a financial surplus to draw on for emergencies, and it used this surplus to give families, businesses, and schools rescue packages four times greater than those in the United States.[29]

In contrast, bailout packages in the United States benefited mainly investors, helping the stock market do well during the first six months of the pandemic but doing little for the millions of Americans who had lost jobs. Because most American workers get medical coverage through employment, unemployment created widespread suffering. As leaders, Chancellor Merkel and President Trump were opposites: while Merkel instituted science-based policies, Trump was anti-science, calling the virus a hoax, pushing unproven, falsified treatments (such as hydroxychloroquine), and empowering random, outlier physicians. Merkel formed alliances with unions and kept factories open, while Trump pushed meat-packing plants and high-school football to stay open without testing. Merkel explained the virus in a way that every German could understand, resulting in widespread support. The support of her citizens saved German hospitals from being overwhelmed. Indeed, given Trump's open hostility to Merkel (he once mocked her dowdy appearance), Germans experienced *Schadenfreude* as the US economy shrank in 2020 by 33 percent, wiping out five years of economic gains, while Germany's shrank by only 10 percent.[30]

Germany did not have the problem that plagued the United States, where Americans had to self-isolate for two weeks not knowing their test results. Results there came back 24 to 48 hours after testing. Citizens will voluntarily self-isolate for two days much more easily than for two weeks. The United States has four times the population of Germany's, but by Halloween, the United States had 24 times the number of cases. Germany spotted infections early, used con-tact tracing well, and had the highest testing-per-capita rate in the world. When in late 2020 Chancellor Merkel announced that she would not seek re-election in 2021, and with upcoming regional elections diluting unity, officials relaxed some restrictions and surges appeared that stressed hospitals. When infections of the highly aggressive B117 variant began in early 2021, Germany tightened its borders with Austria and the Czech Republic.

Alas, the bureaucracy of the European Union (EU) hamstrung Merkel and Germany as a whole with respect to vaccines: the EU bought late, with many conditions, and mainly from AstraZeneca, which did not deliver on time, frus-trating many Germans. The botched rollout of vaccines severely hurt the repu-tation of the EU and vindicated pro-Brexit people in the United Kingdom. The painfully slow rollout of vaccines has meant more lockdowns in Merkel's last months, while rivals plot to be her successor, sometimes currying favor among businesspeople by opposing her policies. The combination of the stealthy rise of the B117 and P1 variants in Germany and close to its borders with the painfully slow rollout of vaccines completely reversed Germany's former reputation as a world leader in controlling SARS2. German children may have been trauma-tized by months-long lockdowns and German seniors could not get vaccinated in any way like their counterparts in the United Kingdom, creating widespread frustration with both Merkel and the EU.[31]

Islands Confront the Virus with Different Models

Island nations with good leaders had unique advantages in fighting pandem-ics. Not all islands had leaders focused on combating the virus (as Britain did), but even those as large as Australia did well when their leaders banned foreign travelers and united the country.

Taiwan immediately suspected that Chinese authorities were untruthful about SARS2, and in January 2020 it banned all travelers from Wuhan, alerting the world to possible dangers. Fifteen months later, and by walling its island against the rest of the world, Taiwan had only 10 Covid deaths and fewer than a thousand infections, allowing citizens to live normally.

South Korea had failed to respond quickly to MERS in 2015 and learned its lesson, creating an excellent system of public health, with capacity for immediate, mass testing.[32] (Because of its hard border on its peninsula with North Korea, South Korea can act like an island nation, exercising great control over entry.) When SARS2 threatened, South Korea closed its borders, ports, and airports. Amazingly, by 2021, South Korea was remarkably successful containing the virus, keeping its economy open, avoiding lockdowns of large cities, and keeping schools open. Early in the pandemic, it teamed up with 28 different agencies to collect data from phones and credit cards of citizens to identify, isolate, and treat those infected or exposed.[33] About 85 percent of South Koreans accepted such loss of their privacy to benefit public health. Like Sweden or Iceland, it has a relatively homogenous population. Almost immediately, South Korean banned cruise ships from docking, started testing everyone, and ramped up production of PPE. It generously supported anyone who had to miss work because of illness and aggressively traced contacts of its first cases.

The country led well in this crisis: it orchestrated cooperation among public health agencies, business, and media; created, distributed and processed test kits quickly for SARS2, testing everyone for free; and rather than testing only the most vulnerable, it tested everyone, thus also performing what epidemiologists called *sentinel testing*, surveying the overall incidence of the virus in a population like a sentinel who watches for approaching dangers. Rather than forcing people to go to emergency rooms and exposing medical staff there to the virus, it created special, drive-through testing sites. Rather than putting the load of treating Covid patients on ordinary hospitals, it created special treatment facilities for Covid. Previous outbreaks had prepared South Koreans for wearing masks in a pandemic. Epidemiologists claim that universal mask-wearing can cut the transmission of SARS2 among compliant people by as much as 89 percent.[34]

All this benefited the maximum number of people in a country that started with thousands of confirmed, unexpected cases. By doing all these things successfully, South Korea controlled the virus without the oppressive lockdowns of China or Italy. It essentially used Focused Protection well. It even kept open its movie theaters. For most of 2020, South Korea enjoyed the praise of the world; even its baseball games resumed. Although it engaged in nothing like China's aggressive quarantine of Wuhan, it did invade the privacy of its citizens in ways that North Americans might resist. That said, in a country of 52 million which suddenly, in January 2020, had thousands of cases with little advance warning, to have less than 100,000 cases by March 2021, and under 1700 deaths, is a great achievement, especially considering how well its economy has fared and how normal life became there throughout 2020.

New Zealand implemented a version of Total, aiming to eliminate the virus entirely inside its islands. On February 3, 2020, it banned travel from China, but on February 26, its first case occurred. On March 15, Prime Minister Jacinda Ardern imposed a mandatory 14-day quarantine on visitors, followed on March 19 by closing its borders to the outside world. On March 25, Ardern instituted a month-long, "Level 4" lockdown: everyone had to stay at home, schools and businesses closed, with only hospitals, groceries, gas stations, and pharmacies open. People could interact only within their families and exercise locally. When they patronized pharmacies or grocery stores, they had to stay six feet apart, wear masks, and wash hands frequently.

New Zealand tested anyone with symptoms, tested vulnerable populations (such as those in nursing homes, prisons, and ethnic Māoris), tested its citizens randomly, and did so for free, quickly identifying clusters of infection and cutting them off from others. In essence, New Zealand modified Total to fit its island nation and democracy. Throughout, Prime Minister Ardern led effectively, telling her nation about the virus, "Our elimination strategy is a sustained approach to keep the virus out, find it, and stamp it out."[35] Her texts were blunt: "This message is for all of New Zealand. We are depending on you.... Where you stay tonight is where you must stay from now on... it is likely level 4 measures will stay in place for a number of weeks."[36]

New Zealand implemented quick, successful contact tracing. From mid-March to mid-August 2020, in an amazing performance in public health, it successfully contacted and quarantined, within four days of exposure, every infected person on its islands, as well as 80 percent of contacts of those exposed to infections, who were also traced and quarantined within four days of exposure.[37] Ardern aimed to eliminate the virus from her islands and by June 8 had done so. Her transparent, clear policies, based on science and communicated publicly, motivated strong acceptance in New Zealanders for wearing masks, distancing, closing bars and businesses, and testing.

A popular prime minister before the pandemic with 84-percent approval, after the pandemic Jacinda Ardern's approval rate soared to 87 percent.[38] In comparison, 74 percent of Canadians approved of Prime Minister Justin Trudeau's handling of the virus, but only 43 percent in France and the United States approved of presidents Emmanuel Macron or Donald Trump. By mid-June, as the virus had infected 4 million in the United States and killed 150,000, New Zealand had had only nine active cases. By August 11, with a population of nearly 5 million, it had gone 100 days without a local transmission.[39]

In the United States, the state most like New Zealand was Vermont, which also aimed to eliminate the virus within its borders. It didn't do that, but in the first 12 months of the pandemic there, it had only 107 deaths, when the rest of the United States had nearly half a million (more on Vermont in Chapter 11).

Although New Zealand received the most publicity, neighboring Australia also did a remarkably good job, employing modified Total. By February 4, 2021, fewer Australians had died (909) than the average daily death rate in Great Britain or the United States.[40] So extremely did Australia pursue elimination that it locked down Perth after one positive case in February. Like Japan and China, it also stranded thousands of its citizens overseas. Unlike Japan and China, it did allow rare foreigners to take in-demand jobs in Australia, but such immigrants had to quarantine in a hotel room for 14 days with monitors in the hallways to guarantee they didn't leave their rooms.[41] Such extreme policies allowed Australians to resume normal lives during the spring of 2021.

Hawaii's governor David Ige told visitors to stay away and shut down travel among its seven inhabited islands. Hawaii even paid for visitors to fly home. It tracked every case with a formidable team of 100 contact tracers.[42] It used flight information to call every person who had visited from China and ordered them to quarantine for two weeks, calling them daily to ensure they quarantined. To those lacking friends or relatives on the island, volunteers delivered groceries and supplies. Hawaii's quarantine was voluntary for those infected and monitored only by phone calls, which stands in contrast to New Zealand's approach of putting infected persons in government-funded hotels. In the fall of 2020, Hawaii required tourists to have a negative test before their boarding their flights. (What those negative tests meant, and their ethical issues, is the subject of Chapter 10.)

Island nations and states cannot depend on much assistance from other countries. So leaders in Taiwan, South Korea, New Zealand, Australia, and Hawaii adopted a "we can sink together or swim together" message. As a result of this message, a sense of togetherness evolved so that citizens did not see restrictions, such as contact tracing, as the product of a hostile government. In its peak week at the end of March 2020, New Zealand had 213 cases, all infected before the lockdown. By the end of April, it had less than a dozen. As its successes grew, New Zealanders took pride in keeping the virus out when it was killing thousands in Italy, and later, hundreds of thousands in the United States.

In Iceland on February 28, 2020, an infected man returned from overseas and contact tracers immediately notified his 56 contacts, but two weeks later, cases there exploded there to between 60 and 100 a day.[43] Iceland then aggressively tested more people per capita than any other country in the world. Importantly, it did not adopt Total. It never required wearing masks. It only shut down bars and hair salons in March and waited until April to teach students at schools and universities virtually and to ban tourists. It adopted Focused Protection.

Iceland's secret weapon was deCODE Genetics, a famous, for-profit genetics company based there, along with the country's previous decision to allow deCODE to sequence the genome of every Icelander to pinpoint genetic diseases. Because Icelanders are homogeneous—almost all descended from a small set of original families—about half of Icelanders are closely related to many other citizens, so genetic privacy is not a big issue to them. As Prime Minister Ardern did in New Zealand, three officials briefed Icelanders every day about cases and control measures. Watching the deaths in Italy, historians reminded Icelanders that smallpox had once killed a quarter of the population.[44] Like Hawaii and New Zealand, Icelanders knew they were stuck on their island and, if infections got out of control again, little outside aid would be coming. At the first real outbreak, deCODE used genetic sequencing machines to identify infected Icelanders and to trace them. By May 17, 2020, deCODE had tested 15.5 percent of Icelanders and had painted a detailed picture of how the virus was spreading.[45] Of great interest to advocates of Focused Protection, Iceland discovered that its children were not spreading the virus to their parents. As the head of deCODE observed, "One of the very interesting things is that, in all our data, there are only two examples where a child infected a parent, but there are lots of examples where parents infected children."[46]

A major destination for tourists, Iceland fared about as well as New Zealand. By March 2021, when New Zealand had experienced about 2,500 cases and 26 deaths, Iceland had about 6,000 cases and 29 deaths.[47] Compared to the United States, Russia, and Brazil, both New Zealand and Iceland did very well.

Canada's Limited Success

Canada did better than the United States in controlling the virus, but not as well as the island nations and states discussed above. On January 25, 2020, a traveler returning from Wuhan brought the first case to Canada, and on March 9, the country had its first death. On March 12, Canada canceled public events with gatherings over 100, eventually reducing them to 50, 10, and then five. University classes went online, and Canada urged retired physicians to come back to help. By March 13, 34,000 Canadians had been tested, four times more than in the United States.

Not everything went well in Canada, however. Early on, Canadian officials gave false assurances about the virus. On January 31, the day when the United States declared a public health emergency, Health Minister Patty Hajdu said, "We're comfortable that we're completely up to date in terms of our approach and what the science says. There is a very low risk to Canadians." Hajdu's low-risk assessment dominated government thinking for too long, making Canada lose a month of preparation. Despite ordering N95 respirators in advance, when the virus hit, Canada lacked enough PPE. Despite recommendations for governments to stockpile PPE following the SARS1 outbreak in Toronto in 2003, Hajdu said the stockpile was never meant for a pandemic, which is undoubtedly true.[48] As with the United States and the WHO, Canadian officials gave contradictory messages about face masks, resulting in confusion. Canadians of Asian descent easily accepted wearing masks, but other Canadians did not.

When Australia banned planes from China, Canada had only four confirmed cases, but rather than doing the same, the Trudeau government argued that travel bans didn't work and even suggested that those proposing them were racist.[49] As late as March 13, Hajdu opposed closing borders. "Canadians think we can stop this at the border," she said. "But what we see is a global pandemic, which means that border measures are highly ineffective and, in some cases, can create harm."[50] Quarantine was also botched. The federal government declined to order the quarantine of travelers returning from China in February because, at the time, public health officials said they lacked the resources to enforce it. A month later, the federal government's emergency order required all returning travelers to quarantine. In response to questions about the decision, Prime Minister Justin Trudeau said the government "did as best we could." On March 21, it closed its border with the United States and banned all foreign visitors.[51] On March 25, Canada finally invoked its Quarantine Act, mandating that all returning persons entering by air, sea, or land must self-isolate for 14 days, excepting essential workers. Anyone arriving in Canada testing positive could not use public transit.

Unlike the United States, where the federal government left states to fight among themselves for PPE and ventilators, the Canadian government ordered 11 million N95 respirator masks and ordered manufacturers to make PPE. Legislation passed giving $2,000 a month to those hurt by Covid from unemployment, sickness, childcare, or care-giving duties. Its federal government paid 75 percent of wages of businesses and charities whose employees had to isolate. Canadians got free testing for Covid.

Canada is very generous with its nursing and retirement homes, but the virus quickly overwhelmed staff there. By May 25, 80 percent of deaths had occurred in such homes. Canada's biggest failure involved its unregulated long-term care homes, which accounted for a disproportionate number of deaths in the country. By April 10, Canada had 10,000 cases. On April 27, after months of hard lockdowns, Ontario released a three-stage plan to re-open its economy. The most important part of that plan required a consistent decline in new cases for three weeks. By April 28, Canada had 50,000 cases. The Canadian government increased by $4 per hour the pay of front-line workers ("hazardous duty pay" in the United States). By August, Canada had tested nearly 4 million people and had 100,000 positive cases.[52] Canada archaically recorded deaths, making doctors fill out and fax paper death certificates to provincial offices, delaying vital statistics needed to get clear pictures of the lethality of the spreading virus. In some provinces, a complete death count might take a year.

Watching what was unfolding in the United States, Canadians mostly unified. Their national medical system dissolved fears about the costs of getting sick. Although provinces shut down restaurants, bars, and businesses, its safety net, like a similar one in Germany, eased the blow and helped Canadians avoid the divisions of the United States. Although at first different provinces responded differently, over months a national "Team Canada" effort emerged that flattened the curve of new cases from a peak of nearly 3,000 a day on May 1 to under a thousand in August. Quebec even re-opened schools in early May. At the same time, the United States saw 50,000 new cases a day. Canadian politicians largely deferred to scientists and did not elevate Covid skeptics. The country did not undermine its own version of the CDC, criticize the WHO, or withdraw funding from it, nor did it politicize facts about the dangers of the virus.

Canada's most populous province, Ontario, imposed severe lockdowns, which included increased powers of police to fine people outside homes. After a surge in cases after Thanksgiving in October 2020, Ontario mandated rolling lockdowns, locking down everyone inside its huge province after Christmas. After another surge in mid-January, the province ordered another lockdown, trying the patience of its weary citizens. By late March 2021, when the United States had 29 million cases and 540,000 deaths, Canada (with a population of about 38 million) had less than 1 million cases and only 22,600 deaths. Overall, Canada did a reasonably good job controlling the unexpected outbreak, showing reasonably good leadership, following science, and consistently messaging.

As in Germany, the agonizingly slow rollout of vaccines frustrated many Canadians. Despite ordering record doses, by February Canada had vaccinated fewer than 2 percent of its citizens, far less than the United Kingdom, United States, or Israel. The inability to make vaccines in Canada didn't help much either, making Canada dependent on importing vaccines from outside. Nor did it help much when officials in Ottawa promised that everyone would be vaccinated by a far-off date—the end of September. The slow roll-out allowed further outbreaks to occur, prompting curfews in Quebec and new restrictions.[53]

India

In 2019, India's Prime Minister Narendra Modi had encouraged Hindu tribalism, scapegoated Muslims, and pushed citizenship laws that discriminated against Muslims, causing protests. When the virus hit, malicious posts on social media by Hindus blamed Muslims for the virus, inflaming tensions. In November 2016, to fight corruption, because bribes had been paid with bags of paper money, Modi gave only four hours' notice before eliminating small-denomination paper currency.[54] His actions severely damaged the economy, a damage he hoped would last only a year. He intended to create a modern economy without bribes and where taxes were paid.

But Modi didn't know a pandemic loomed on the horizon. When SARS2 hit

India in April 2020, again giving only four hours' notice, Modi adopted Intermittent Lockdown, closing almost everything in India, forcing tens of millions to leave the cities where they worked and to take their families to their ancestral villages, where their elderly relatives still lived. Realizing laborers had no money to return to their ancestral villages, the Modi government created 4,621 "Shramik Specials" ("Shramik in Hindi means "laborer"), trains that carried laborers home, many riding a thousand miles on 24-hour-long rides in non-air-conditioned cars where poor laborers rode packed together like subway riders at rush hour.[55] Instead of containing the virus, Modi created a gigantic amplification system, such that in a few months, India's rate of infection soared from a few hundred thousand to 8 million, rivaling the United States. By the end of 2020, India's caseload surpassed 10 million, the second-highest in the world.

The misery inflicted by the crash of India's economy from the double hits described above impoverished India's hundreds of millions of poor people more than anything the virus could have done. Before the pandemic, India had lifted hundreds of millions from poverty, and its economy had been growing, but over the three months of its lockdown in 2020, it lost one-quarter of its GNP, the worst of any economy in the world. The collapse of India's economy created untold misery for India's poor.[56] In the northern state of Punjab, thousands of farmers, overextended in debt, and—when markets collapsed—unable to sell their crops, committed suicide. In 2019, 10,281 farmers killed themselves, and in 2020, due to the pandemic, that number jumped to 30,000.[57] And in addition to those who killed themselves, thousands more suffered from homelessness or hunger.

By that fall, doom had spread across India, and families were forced to sell dowry gold, unthinkable before the pandemic. Indian writer Arundhati Roy said, "The engine [of the economy] has been smashed. The ability to survive has been smashed. And the pieces are all up in the air. You don't know where they are going to fall or how they are going to fall."[58] Meanwhile, Modi pursued market reforms, including a controversial proposal for India's 146 million farms, which led to mass public protests by farmers—protests that further spread the virus.[59]

In mid-May 2021, SARS2 was spreading faster in India than in any country in the world, creating over 300,000 new cases a day. Already, India had the fourth-highest number of Covid deaths in the world (172,000), and its surge in new daily cases was sure to push the number much higher in the future. In retrospect, if Modi had only adopted Focused Protection and had not eliminated paper currency, India would be in far better shape today. Of course, hindsight is always perfect.

Other Developing Economies

Brazil's president, Jair Bolsonaro, took his cues from Donald Trump, downplaying the virus, refusing to wear a mask in public, and promoting hydroxychloroquine. By mid-August 2020, Brazil had 100,000 deaths as the virus spread up the Amazon River basin and slew 1,000 Brazilians a day.[60] By mid-May 2021, the country had over 15 million cases and 432,000 deaths, with a daily Covid death rate surpassing the United States. So widespread were infections in the Brazilian Amazon city of Manaus that a new variant emerged, P1, which quickly overwhelmed the original SARS2 virus and then spread to Europe and North America, which demonstrates the dangers to richer countries of abandoning poorer countries. By banding together to fight global pandemics, all countries benefit in preventing the emergence of new and dangerous variants.

Mexico's president, Manuel Obrador, like Bolsonaro, took a harsh attitude to the virus, even though he became infected himself. It took a few months for the virus to penetrate developing Mexico and Ecuador, but once it entered, it fueled waves of infection.[61] Obrador resisted testing, earning praise from Donald Trump, who said, "I want to do what Mexico does. They don't give you a test till you get to the emergency room and you're vomiting."[62] By May 2021, Mexico had the fourth-highest number of deaths, behind India, Brazil, and the US, with 220,000 dead.[63]

INTERMITTENT LOCKDOWNS, DENIAL, AND THE AMERICAN CONFUSION

Between December 15, 2019, and January 15, 2020, thousands of people flew from Wuhan to London and Germany, and over 900 flew to New York City, some of them carrying SARS2. Not until January 23 did the United States ban all flights from China, when SARS2 had already arrived in many American cities.

Former president Trump seems to have believed that the United States would fare best with an open economy, so he did not try to contain the virus. In January, some thought that SARS2 might disappear the way MERS did in 2015, Swine flu gradually did in 2009, SARS1 did in 2003, and Swine flu did in 1976, possibly because the coming warm summer months might weaken it. For complex reasons that will be debated for decades (see Chapter 12), the Trump administration did not take seriously what was happening in Wuhan and Italy. The administration did not ban flights from China until February 3, 2020. By that time, 1,300 flights from China had arrived at 17 US airports, carrying over 430,000 people. Thousands of other international flights allowed millions of people to enter the United States between January and April.[64]

If you favor Total, the United States and Canada made many mistakes, but even if you favor Focused Protection, the United States failed to do the normal, easy measures that would have reduced the virus's spread, such as universal wearing of masks, physical distancing, and banning large crowds. In some ways, the first months of the American response was Swedish. As will be explored in the next chapter about the distribution of ventilators and in Chapter 7 about the distribution of vaccines, President Trump barely had a plan for stopping the virus. Although they did not know it by this name, American businessmen favored the Swedish approach, especially owners of bars, restaurants, gyms, movie theaters, casinos, and theme parks, all of which were shut down in Italy and in island democracies. And although they did not know it by this name either, many parents favored the milder Focused Protection, especially when they learned that the virus killed few children and that most children won't even get sick.

On March 11, as data suggested infections coming to New York from Europe, the Trump administration banned foreign nationals on flights from Europe, not the United Kingdom, after March 13. Sensing other imminent restrictions, Americans in Europe immediately scrambled to return home, jamming airports in Atlanta and New York City with large crowds, few wearing masks, and jostling each other in crowded lines close together for hours. Because of the uncoordinated, chaotic way in which the government announced the ban, these airports became amplification systems. (A similar mistake occurred when the Trump administration disregarded the CDC's strenuous advice not to fly asymptomatic Americans home from the Diamond Princess cruise ship on the same plane with infected Americans.) Neither the CDC nor Atlanta authorities had been consulted as to how to make things safe for returning Americans. In eight days, because of returning Americans and because of people already infected, cases in the United States jumped from one hundred to a thousand.[65]

On January 19, in Snohomish County in Washington state, an American who had returned four days earlier from Wuhan tested positive for SARS2.[66] Shortly thereafter, a nursing home in King County in the same state reported a cluster of cases. Based on genetic tests of 7,000 blood samples donated by Americans the month before, SARS2 had entered the United States as early as December 13, 2019 (samples showed antibodies to coronaviruses in 106 cases, and specific antibodies to SARS2 in one, maybe two, samples).[67]

On March 2, New Rochelle, a suburb north of New York City, experienced a cluster of cases centered on a Jewish lawyer and his synagogue. Governor Andrew Cuomo instituted an aggressive containment zone around it, hoping to flatten the curve of new infections. Unknown to the governor, a thousand New Yorkers had likely already been infected by using New York City's massive subway, bus, and train systems, which supported nearly four billion rides a year, with rush hours packing riders close together.

By April 2, of the 200,000 cases in the United States, 84,000 crested in New York. Ambulances bringing sick Covid patients to emergency rooms howled through the night in the five boroughs, causing massive anxiety. Soon, over a thousand Americans died in just one day.[68] To house overflows, the Army Corps of Engineers built a field hospital in the Javits Convention Center, and the Navy's *Comfort* docked in New York harbor. Many Covid patients required intensive care and ventilators, which became scarce, and bioethicists debated how to distribute them.

Governor Cuomo ordered a hard lockdown, closing most of New York City and the state of New York. Like New Zealand's Prime Minister Ardern, he held informative, daily press briefings, pleading for a national response and for help, feuding with President Trump, who urged keeping businesses and schools to stay open. On March 21, Trump had announced a "tough two weeks ahead" as infections continued to spike. He appointed a Corona Task Force to manage the federal government's response to the virus, headed by Vice-President Mike Pence, which announced a 30-day plan to overcome the virus. Cities and states everywhere, from California to Alabama, restricted public gatherings, closing bars and restaurants, but it was too late: by the next week, the United States led the world in cases, with 100,000. After months of intensive care, many doctors and nurses in New York City were depressed and burned out; two female physicians in New York City caring for Covid patients committed suicide. Through strenuous efforts and Cuomo's leadership, New York eventually flattened its curve.

A huge problem in the United States was that, unlike other developed countries, tests took too long to give results. South Korea and Italy developed quick, immediate tests, but in the United States, which perceived itself technologically superior to most nations, test results often took a week or more to receive, sometimes as long as 16 days. It took eight days for the mayor of Atlanta, Keisha Lance Bottoms, to learn of her positive result, and six days for the son of the president's chief of staff. Given that many people only start to think about getting a test when they have symptoms, and given that many wait hours or even days in drive-throughs to get tested, the delay in reporting results gave the virus a week or more to spread when infected people didn't know they were infecting others (by the time she learned she was infected, three people in Mayor Bottoms's family had also been infected). Such problems in testing made contact tracing and self-quarantining difficult. (These problems are explored in Chapter 10.)

A continuing problem was lack of standardization of reporting across states. Critics charged the CDC with failure to correct the hodge podge ways of reporting infections and deaths by hospitals, nursing homes, factories, and prisons.[69] Without good data, Michael Osterholm, director of the Center for Disease Research in Minnesota, correctly complained, "How do you know if you're succeeding or failing?"[70]

Throughout this pandemic, Dr. Anthony Fauci, the director of the National Institute of Allergy and Infectious Disease since 1984, became the authority most Americans trusted. Ironically, Fauci had been vilified in the first years of AIDS for his reluctance to fast-track anti-HIV drugs. To his credit, Fauci listened to activists and gave them a voice at the table. As one writer noted in 2020, looking back to the early days of HIV/AIDS:

Most notably, he dramatically loosened HIV-drug clinical trial requirements so that a far greater number of desperate patients could try new compounds (an approach called "parallel tracking"), expanded research on HIV/AIDS and its treatment in underrepresented women and/or people of color, and gave activists and people living with HIV seats at the table of the planning committee of the AIDS Clinical Trials Group (ACTG). Fauci also played a key role in getting the federal research apparatus to incorporate those recommendations, in what amounted to perhaps the first time that federal health bureaucrats acceded almost fully to community and activist demands.[71]

Activists eventually reconciled with Fauci, calling him "the only true and great hero" among government officials in the AIDS crisis.[72]

One of the worst moments of the Trump era occurred when the President announced on national television that a drug used to treat malaria, hydroxychloroquine, could treat Covid. In May, he shocked his medical advisors by similarly suggesting on national television that scientists should investigate whether household bleach or ultraviolet light could "clean the system of the virus." In the same month, he told the press that he himself had been taking hydroxychloroquine to ward off the virus. (It did not help, as he eventually became infected). On May 15, he announced Operation Warp Speed, a multi-billion-dollar project to create vaccines for Covid, promised before the end of 2020 and, he hoped, before the November election. National leaders of vaccine research worried that the vaccine's safety would not be thoroughly tested.[73] So widespread was this worry that nearly half of Americans said they would not be the first to take such a vaccine.[74]

On Memorial Day in May 2020, many states re-opened beaches, which became crowded with happy revelers at the end of the shutdowns. These amplification systems soon spiked infections in Florida, Texas, and other parts of the South, overwhelming hospitals there by mid-July and demoralizing medical professionals who risked their lives in caring for irresponsible citizens. Such "Covid-deniers" created ethical quandaries in the ICU when they denied they had Covid, declined helpful drugs, and refused to mend their ways.

In October 2020, editors of the *New England Journal of Medicine* issued a rare political condemnation just before the presidential election, breaking with a two-century tradition of avoiding endorsements in elections:

Why has the United States handled this pandemic so badly? We have failed at almost every step. We had ample warning, but when the disease first arrived, we were incapable of testing effectively and couldn't provide even the most basic personal protective equipment to health care workers and the general public. And we continue to be way behind the curve in testing. While the absolute numbers of tests have increased substantially, the more useful metric is the number of tests performed per infected person, a rate that puts us far down the international list, below such places as Kazakhstan, Zimbabwe, and Ethiopia, countries that cannot boast the biomedical infrastructure or the manufacturing capacity that we have. Moreover, a lack of emphasis on developing capacity has meant that U.S. test results are often long delayed, rendering the results useless for disease control.[75]

The spring of 2021 seemed to vindicate Governor DeSantis's actions in Florida, which had many vulnerable seniors but a morality rate 50 percent lower than New York. Moreover, New York's hard lockdowns and strict mitigation efforts severely hurt businesses, while Florida remained largely open and prospered.[76] DeSantis had also participated in a roundtable discussion with the co-authors of the Great Barrington Declaration, the leading advocates of Focused Protection.

FINAL NOTE

Measuring the costs and harms of each model is difficult, in part because accurate statistics take years to accumulate and in part because interpretations can be political. Because some citizens had no choice about the model under which they lived, passions erupted about decisions to adopt a particular model. Some people hated both Total and Intermittent Lockdown, feeling that those who supported them were bad people, while others despised the Swedish approach, also implying that bad people adopted it. In the end, perhaps those who adopted different models simply held different philosophical positions about how to fight pandemics.

One thing is clear: if the only goal was to squash the virus, the countries that did best quickly banned incoming travel (even for returning citizens), contained outbreaks, mandated physical distancing and mask-wearing, aggressively contact-traced and monitored those quarantined, closed restaurants, bars, and gyms, banned social gatherings, and did not quickly re-open, all while clearly and consistently telling citizens what was occurring and why.

FURTHER READING

de Waal, Alex, and Paul Richards. "Coronavirus: Why Lockdowns May Not Be the Answer in Africa." BBC News. 14 April 2020.

"Great Barrington Declaration." https://gbdeclaration.org/.

Hessler, Peter. "The Sealed City." New Yorker. 12 October 2020.

McNeil, Donald. "To Take on the Coronavirus, Go Medieval on It." New York Times. 28 February 2020.

Oldstone, Michael. Viruses, Plagues and History. Oxford: Oxford University Press, 2010.

Smart, Benjamin, Alex Broadbent, and Herkulaas Combrink. "Lockdown Didn't Work in South Africa: Why It Shouldn't Happen Again." The Conversation. 15 October 2020.

CHAPTER 5
WHO SHOULD LIVE WHEN NOT ALL CAN?

"We don't want a situation where we're putting bedside physicians in the position of making decisions patient by patient," said Felicia Cohn, clinical professor of bioethics at the UC Irvine School of Medicine.[1] When the virus hit northern Italy hard in the months before it hit New York, a doctor lamented, "We have to decide who must die and whom we shall keep alive."[2]

This chapter discusses ethical issues in distributing scarce medical resources during the Covid surge in New York City in the spring of 2020, when hospitals sometimes lacked enough ventilators, machines that assist breathing. Such allocation problems can be handled in many different ways. One way is to anticipate imminent problems of distribution and try to prevent them. For example, in New York City during the surge, some nursing homes refused to accept the return of Covid patients who had been at their facilities. Because they were full, other hospitals re-directed ambulances to other emergency rooms. Of course, these individual decisions by hospitals do not reflect an overall plan, which would have been good to have.

ETHICAL THEORIES AS GUIDES

Utilitarianism

Utilitarianism, founded by Jeremy Bentham and John Stuart Mill in England in the early nineteenth century as a social reform movement, contrasted with moralities based on religious founders or the prevailing social order in England, which emphasized class and hereditary privilege. The most basic question in ethical theory asks, "What, if anything, makes an act right?," to which utilitarianism answers, "The greatest good for the greatest number of beings."

Utilitarianism contains three parts: (1) its *maximization principle*: the greatest good for the greatest number of beings must be sought; (2) its *consequentialist mandate*: actual consequences to beings matter, not just good motives or good character; (3) a *definition of "good" and "beings"*: the adjective "good" in "good consequences" must have some measure, as well as "beings." Bentham was a hedonic utilitarian, measuring good in terms of pleasure and pain; hence, *hedonic utilitarianism* defines right acts as producing the greatest amount of pleasure for the greatest number of beings.

To its critics, utilitarianism contains many problems, among them the following: What counts as a "being" in the "greatest number of beings"? Do animals count? Bentham thought so, as do modern utilitarians such as Peter Singer. Next, what is the scope of the principle? Just my hospital? My region? My nation? The globe? Finally, the maximization problem dictates actions that conflict with other moral theories, such as Kantian ethics, because it seems to endorse the sacrifice of the one for the good of the many. Despite these problems, utilitarianism offers a useful, practical theory for fields as different as economics and public health. Its most famous modern champion is Australian bioethicist Peter Singer, whose early book *Animal Liberation* (1975) sparked the modern movement of Animal Rights and moral vegetarianism, and who also influenced Effective Altruism, a movement dedicated to guiding charitable giving with rigorous empirical research.[3]

With respect to Covid, in the allocation of ventilators and admission to intensive care units, utilitarianism directs us to save as many lives as possible through admissions to the emergency room, if necessary by triage. In mass disaster, utilitarianism not only permits triage but requires it. Although it seems harsh to abandon someone who is dying, such triage is pro-life because its goal is to maximize lives saved. During pandemics, no physician or hospital during a pandemic can take care of all needy patients. Understanding that, some hospitals create *triage officers*, people charged with deciding whom to admit.

Triage comes from the French word meaning sorting or picking, and it has since come to mean sorting into groups. Such sorting started to be known by that name when used by the French physician Dominique Larrey, a surgeon during Napoleon's campaign in Egypt and Syria at the turn of the nineteenth century, which resulted in heavy casualties.[4] Larrey divided the battlefield's wounded into three groups regardless of rank: those who would be unlikely to live, regardless of what care they would receive, those who would live without medical intervention, and those for whom medical intervention could turn imminent death to life. He employed horse-drawn ambulances to shuttle those in the last group to field hospitals; the others, he stoically left behind.

Authorities employed triage in 2017 after a lone gunman in a Las Vegas casino-hotel shot many patrons celebrating at a music festival below his hotel room. After the meltdowns of the Chernobyl and Fukushima nuclear reactors, authorities also used triage. In utilitarian ethics, these triage situations are called *lifeboat cases*. Consider a ship's officer commanding a lifeboat after the sinking of the ocean liner *Titanic*. Scores of desperate passengers are swimming in lethally cold waters attempting to board a boat that can hold only a fraction of them. If the officer lets in too many people, his boat will sink. Once filled to capacity, he cannot endanger the lives of those inside by letting others come aboard, so he must encourage those already aboard to help him resist entry of others. At worst, he must use an oar to hit people trying to get in.

Variations of lifeboat cases have occurred in reality, and ethicists have imagined many more. Suppose the lifeboat floats in the middle of the Pacific Ocean with no help likely on the way. The officer sees strong young people clinging to debris around the lifeboat, which holds some frail seniors. Should they allow only strong rowers inside and reject the elders, with a long trip to land ahead? And with a storm approaching, a crew of strong, young rowers gives all on board the best chance of surviving.

Worldwide, triage can be applied to nations or regions. Consider the worldwide fight to stop the spread of AIDS. In 2008, the United States committed $48 billion for five years to combat the spread of HIV around the globe.[5] Thailand then did an amazing job fighting AIDS, as did Brazil, both offering free testing, free condoms, and educational messages. Uganda dropped its overall rate of HIV infection by half across the country as a whole and by two-thirds among urban, pregnant women. But in South Africa, in 1999 President Thabo Mbeki denied that AIDS was real, and his townships experienced some of the world's highest rates of HIV infection. Although it sounds harsh, if $1 million could prevent a thousand young Ugandan women from getting infected, and if the same money spent in South Africa had no effect because of Mbeki's denialism, shouldn't the money be spent in Uganda? The world faced a similar problem in 2021 when the late Tanzanian president John Magufuli announced that his country would reject Covid vaccines and instead use an herbal cocktail of garlic, lemon juice, and ginger to cure the virus.[6]

Sadly, sometimes a country has such vast problems that no amount of humanitarian aid can save its peoples. Angola, Eritrea, Libya, Iraq, Yemen, Somalia, and Haiti may be failed states. To keep pouring money into them for triage is like letting more and more people into the lifeboat until it sinks.

Care Ethics

During the 1980s, feminist psychologists, philosophers, and education professors, especially Carol Gilligan, decided that male philosophers had created traditional ethical theories that were too abstract, too intellectual, and too false with respect to the experience of women. They called their own resulting theory care ethics (or the ethics of care). Subsequent feminist theorists explored family relationships and virtues of caring, nurturing, trust, intimate friendship, bonding, and love. Rather than focusing on atomistic individuals, care ethics emphasizes the family, which bioethical analysis sometimes previously ignored.

According to this theory, we want physicians to treat people within their *circle of concern*. Within a hospital unit, we want nurses to feel for patients under their supervision. Care ethics recognizes that, in the real world or the family or hospital, care is a limited resource. Although it may sound harsh, it's not realistic for nurses to be concerned with a thousand dying patients in Yemen. That's not their job, and besides, in the Covid world, they're already exhausted from nursing those near them.

Critics say that care ethics does not tell us how to treat people we do not know or, more simply, those we do not care about. Nurses often meet patients as strangers. In other words, if our ability to care diminishes as we expand our "circle of concern" from family to neighbors to colleagues to region, one wonders whether care ethics can guide public policy. More important, how will it adjudicate the inevitable conflicts between all the "circles of concern" over access to scarce resources? Consider Nurse Jones, who has never met George and Brianna, two 20-year-olds in the ER, and she only recently started taking care of 85-year-old Sam in the ICU. Should she maximally treat Sam and ignore George and Brianna?

Dissenting feminists believe that care ethics reinforces stereotypes of gender, such as the notion that women, not men, care about the family and those near them. As one wit said, "The ethics of care screams, 'Mommy!'" Nor does it tell us how to resolve conflicts among people we care about, such as when a physician must choose between checking on a patient and being with her own daughter at childbirth. In reply, some care bioethicists do address issues far beyond the family, such as the plight of HIV-infected women around the world or female circumcision in Africa. Overall, care ethics may correct legalistic reasoning or abstract, quantitative calculations in bioethics.

Nevertheless, care ethics clearly directs us to first take care of our families, our friends, and our colleagues at work. In the movie *Contagion*, Laurence Fishburne plays a CDC doctor, Ellis Cheever, who acquires a successful vaccine that only a few will get. Although he does not inject himself, he does violate the national lottery and gives it to his wife. Care ethics would endorse his action. I discuss care ethics more below when dealing with organ allocation and the rule of rescue.

Kantian Ethics

Immanuel Kant, the chief moral thinker of the Enlightenment, answers the question, "What makes an act right?" differently than either proponents of utilitarianism or care ethics. For Kant, the only true criterion of moral goodness is wanting to do the right thing, which he defined as having a *good will*. Having a good will means desiring the right things and possessing the right motives or intentions. It is Kant's name for moral virtue.

Kant, a supreme rationalist, believed that humans could aspire to moral greatness, although they usually failed. To so aspire, they must act so that the rule or maxim under which they act can be *universalized*, that is, can be willed under which to act by all similar, rational people. He called the obligation to act this way the *categorical imperative*. He also gave an alternative version: "Always act to treat people as absolute ends-in-themselves, never as mere means." Kant's requirement of universalizability implies transparency, which may matter greatly when everyone wants something that everyone cannot have, such as a scarce vaccine. For life-and-death decisions, Kant requires that everyone should be treated equally. That is the only way to preserve equal moral worth and to treat people as "ends in themselves."

What that means may be best understood in contrast. Treating everyone the same means not treating your family and friends first. It means not judging that some are more valuable than others. More controversially, it means not judging that giving Jones 20 years of future life outweighs giving 90-year-old Smith two more years. The latter view is implied by utilitarianism. To Kant, utilitarianism implies that surgeons should cut up a homeless young man without family and transplant his organs to save several needy patients. But taking innocent human life is always wrong for Kant, even to save lives of others. The end of "more lives saved" does not justify the means of murder.

In the lifeboat, Kant's best answer is to have a lottery about who gets to stay. For a new, successful vaccine, Kantian ethics favors a lottery that treats everyone with equal moral worth. For Kant, it is always wrong to use one person to benefit another. It makes no difference that the people are children in the same family or relatives. People should never be treated *as a mere means* for the welfare of others. As we will see in our examination of a vaccine trial in the Philippines for Dengue fever, for Kant, it is also wrong for a parent to use one child to save another. Once one child's health can be sacrificed to save another, one has embarked on a kind of reasoning that leads to dark corners.

Consider what has happened in transplant medicine. In 1954, from a Kantian perspective an ethical bright line was wrongly crossed, allowing one twin to donate a kidney to save another, opening the door to intra-family kidney, lung, and liver transplants, which now have become normal, where relatives often feel pressure to "donate."[7] If one follows the path of this reasoning, one arrives at a place that may be considered a *reductio ad absurdum* conclusion. Consider the tragic situation where a single mother is dying of liver disease and the only compatible possible "donor" is her eight-year-old son. Is it justified to take part of the son's liver to try to save the mother? Doing so unquestionably harms the son, although it probably won't kill him or leave him with a lifelong disability. But the operation *could do so*, and that is the ethical problem. Once we cross this line, will all children be seen as solid organ resources for their dying parents?

Consider also the tragic situation where parents have two children dying, both of whom need organ transplants, as well as a healthy third child who is a compatible organ donor. In this situation, does not utilitarian or cost-benefit reasoning justify killing the one healthy child to save the dying two? And what if the tragedy is even greater? Suppose an explosion has occurred, injuring a family of seven who will die unless one healthy child not present at the explosion is sacrificed to save them. Even though we know that saving seven lives is good, and that the good of two outweighs the good of one, Kant believes that it is absolutely wrong to act in this way. Killing innocent children is intrinsically wrong, even to save other innocent children. This act cannot be universalized as a maxim for all humans to act on. As philosopher Elizabeth Anscombe said of President Harry Truman's decision to drop atomic bombs, *some things may not be done, no matter what.*[8]

For Kant, utilitarian cost–benefit reasoning leads us down a dark path that may have a worthy goal at the first stop but can empower other travelers to act similarly for less worthy goals. For Kant, once we accept this utilitarian framework that one person can be harmed to save others, *a corruption of reasoning* develops, leading us down a conceptual slippery slope, possibly allowing physicians to go from harming one child to *save* another's life to harming one child to merely *benefit* another.

Given the realities of life's scarcities, Kantian ethics can be tweaked to fit circumstances. It might favor making exceptions to a lottery for workers constantly exposed to SARS2, because if they don't stay healthy, who will take care of infected patients? After they are inoculated, then a lottery could occur for everyone else. In the same way, Kant might favor giving everyone a week in the ICU and then if things go badly for Smith, removing Smith in favor of someone else. The universalized maxim would be, "Everyone gets a chance at the ICU bed for a week." That policy treats everyone the same and avoids the distasteful outcomes of first-come, first-served, where one very ill patient occupies the ICU room for several months while others die waiting.

Rawlsian Justice and the Most Vulnerable

The major theory of justice of the twentieth century came from philosopher John Rawls, who combined elements of Kantian ethics with social contract theory to argue for basic structures of a just society.[9] Rawls had people choose under *a veil of ignorance* about personal characteristics of ourselves such as looks, race, gender, sexual orientation, wealth, or class. This intellectual tool forces us to put ourselves in the place of those less fortunate, in essence forcing us to choose basic structures of society through the lens of the Golden Rule, so Rawls's theory is both Kantian and within the traditions of the major Western religions. His theory also resonates with Hinduism, especially its belief that what one does in this life creates karma that determines one's place in the next, or with Stoicism ("What we do in life, echoes in eternity"[10]).

Under such a veil of ignorance, Rawls famously argued that citizens would opt, first, for maximal equal liberty for each of them, compatible with similar liberty for others, and second, for his difference principle, the idea that inequalities were justified only if they benefited the least-well-off groups. As such, Rawls argued that we would choose to make that position as good as possible. We would choose a bottom-up rather than a trickle-down approach.

Rawls is Kantian in several senses. First, he believes we have the capacity in ethics to think and act rationally. Second, because his veil of ignorance forces us to act for the good of the least well-off group, it forces us to act under the Golden Rule. In that sense, it resembles Kant's requirement of universalizable maxims. Rawls differs from Kant in appealing to self-interest in the social contract, which Kant would abhor. Let's take an example. With as many as 30 million Americans lacking medical coverage, a just society would not organize medical finance with physicians making high incomes. Single-payer systems, such as those enjoyed by Canadians or New Zealanders, come closer to the Rawlsian ideal. What is that ideal? It is that getting injured or sick is bad luck that no one can predict in advance, and when it occurs, the lack of ability to pay for medical treatment shouldn't be an added harm. Having a national system of medical coverage operationalizes the idea that "we're all in this together." For Rawls, medicine should not be a license for specialists to become millionaires but should be a system to care for the medically vulnerable. The opposite is the system of private medical coverage in the United States that operates to profit by selling coverage to those who least need it and by denying it to those who do.

To whom, then, would Rawls give scarce ventilators or ICU rooms? It would not necessarily be to those most vulnerable to die from Covid, because some of them might be dying anyway. Instead, it would be those at the bottom of society who are most unfairly exposed to SARS2, such as poorly paid workers in nursing homes, who contract the virus at a high rate. Another group would be prisoners and undocumented workers held in crowded detention centers. Another group would be workers in meat-packing plants such as the 3,700 workers at the Smithfield ham plant in Sioux Falls, South Dakota, which processes 20,000 hogs a day and where the virus has infected over 1,300 workers and killed at least four.[11]

Final Note about Ethical Theories

Some rationality must be introduced into medical systems for allocating scarce resources, be those resources hearts or ventilators, livers or ICU rooms. To throw everything into the first patient admitted to the hospital (who also might happen to be the richest and most socially connected) will waste many resources. Our survey of ethical theories has also showed that use of such theories will not provide easy answers to dilemmas of the allocation of medical resources created by the SARS2 pandemic. The great historian of ethics Alasdair MacIntyre, in his *Short History of Ethics*, compared our moral intuitions today to the debris left on the seas after a great naval battle between the several warships of two countries, with each warship representing an ethical theory—such as Kantian ethics, contractarianism, utilitarianism, care ethics, or virtue ethics—and now we are left with chunks and parts of each destroyed ship, all left floating and interspersed together, none whole and livable, analogous to the conflicting ethical intuitions that we've inherited from past ethical traditions and which conflict inside us in different cases.[12]

There are still those who have been raised in ethical traditions that give them definitive answers about how to live, as in Judaism, various branches of Islam, and some Christian traditions, such as Latter-day Saints. But most of us have inherited multiple beliefs or feelings from differing traditions: we are Greek perfectionists in watching the Olympics, Lockean champions of property rights when our vehicles are stolen, and utilitarians on committees trying to do the most good. That we have no easy way to resolve conflicting beliefs does not make our situation hopeless, however. There is power in understanding where our beliefs come from and their backgrounds in ethical theories. There is power in studying how others have solved similar conflicts. Moreover, simply because some beliefs conflict with each other does not mean there are not better and worse solutions to those conflicts. Being reasonable, appreciating evidence, showing compassion to the vulnerable—all these have value in the modern world, especially during pandemics.

HISTORICAL BACKGROUND: THE GOD COMMITTEE AND SOCIAL WORTH

Issues of distributive justice raised by the Covid pandemic arose in 1962 with the "God Committee" in Seattle, Washington, infamous in bioethics for adopting a *social worth criterion* of who received a then-scarce, experimental hemodialysis machine. Created to avoid the biases of care ethics, the God Committee removed the burden of moral decision making from physicians, who each wanted their own patients to be dialyzed and live. The committee of seven consisted of a minister, a lawyer, a housewife, a labor leader, a state government official, a banker, and a surgeon. Two physicians familiar with dialysis screened applicants for medical unsuitability. The committee worked anonymously and never met candidates.[13]

The committee first limited candidates to residents of the state of Washington who were under 45; and these candidates had to be able to afford dialysis or have insurance that covered it. Almost immediately, too many patients applied, and additional criteria became necessary. Famously, the committee then considered personal characteristics such as employment, children, education, motivation, achievements, and promise of helping others—criteria somewhat like those used by committees to admit students to medical school. The committee eventually asked for analyses of a candidate's abilities to tolerate anxiety and to manage medical care independently; it considered whether a candidate had previously used symptoms to get attention. It evaluated the personality and personal merit of the candidate and the family's support for the relative on dialysis. Elderly curmudgeons without siblings or children fared badly.

Law professors and journalists pummeled the committee for implying that some patients deserved dialysis more than others. Its social worth criteria violated the idea in Kantian ethics of equal moral worth. But care ethics had little to criticize when the committee prioritized a young single mother with three children over an elderly bachelor. And if the young mother rarely drank alcohol but the elderly bachelor drank excessively, few would disagree that the mother would better keep her appointments and be more likely to do well on dialysis.

When a reporter outed the God Committee in a prominent magazine's cover story, the US Congress could not agree on criteria of just allocation, so it went on a spending spree and guaranteed every American, in the End Stage Renal Disease Act, to a right, first, to dialysis, and later to a kidney transplant—all at federal expense. In this way, politicians avoided any national discussion about who should receive artificial or transplanted kidneys. Although no such national coverage exists for Americans for heart, liver, bone marrow, skin, or face transplants, they do enjoy a national right to dialysis and kidney transplants.

A RELEVANT DIGRESSION: "SICKEST FIRST" ALLOCATION AND UNOS

Like utilitarianism, care ethics can go awry. One such case concerns the *sickest first criterion* that the United Network for Organ Sharing (UNOS) uses to distribute hearts and livers in the United States. According to this criterion, those who have waited the longest or who are closest to death get priority for receiving a suddenly available heart or liver. This standard satisfied the families of patients waiting for such transplants. But utilitarians disagree. Because underlying diseases have pushed these patients near to death, and because these organs could have gone to younger, healthier patients, this criterion does not maximize lived years per transplanted organ. Care ethics enters the picture here because the patients who have been waiting for a long time for organs, sometimes years, have bonded to staff and developed strong relationships with them. Patients awaiting transplants enter the "circle of concern" of staff and become almost like family. Surgeons feel that, after such a long relationship, to give an organ to a newly arrived stranger is tantamount to abandoning their long-time patients.

Such intensity of relationships leads to a *reductio ad absurdum* in allocation of scarce organs, where the same identified patient can get organ after organ while others get none. In one case, 11-year old Danny Canal received a total 12 organs, four organs in each of three different times. This is not an isolated case, as many re-transplants occur. But why did Danny get so many while others waiting never got one? One answer is that his father knew how to work the system. A better answer is that the surgical team liked this cute white kid and hated to see him die. In bioethics, this is called the *rule of rescue*. Danny's surgeons gave him more and more organs because they *cared* about him, heroically and finally saving him, but at great cost to strangers who died because these organs did not go to them. But to utilitarians, this is an absurd waste of organs. Kant would agree, favoring the maxim, "Everyone gets a chance at one organ before anyone gets two organs." In essence, two impartial theories, Kantianism and utilitarianism, vie against the "partialist" theory of care ethics.

In our Covid world, a similarly wasteful situation would be that the first patients admitted to the hospital get maximal resources—ICU beds, ventilators, antibody treatment, and new drugs—but those in the waiting room get nothing. This would be like the triage officer on a scene of mass casualties putting people in ambulances based on who was on the ground closest to him, regardless of their condition.

ENTER BIOETHICISTS

An enormous amount of work in bioethics occurred before the Covid pandemic. One famous article by philosopher Nicholas Rescher in 1969 outlined selection criteria for allocating dialysis machines.[14] He advocated awarding points according to the relative likelihood of success, expectance of future life, family role (e.g., a single mother with three children), and (controversially) past and future services to society. For patients whose total scores tied, Rescher advocated a lottery. In real life, physicians and others do not feel comfortable making judgments about past and future contributions to society. To say the radiologist deserves the kidney more than the housekeeper seems to violate Kant's principle of equal moral worth; besides, the radiologist may be a selfish jerk and the housekeeper, a saint.

Bioethicist-physician Ezekiel Emanuel emerged as a leader during the pandemic, both on cable television and in various op-ed essays. He had previously helped craft the 2010 Patient Care and Affordable Care Act (aka "Obamacare") when his brother Rahm served as White House chief of staff until 2010 (and then as mayor of Chicago until 2019). An article by Emanuel summarized several views about allocating scarce medical resources, including sickest first, a lottery, and social worth. He sided with utilitarianism, concluding that the highest priority should be to "save the most lives" and most "life years."[15] For hospitals with Covid patients making decisions with scarce resources, Emanuel advocates *maximizing life-years saved.*

"Disability-adjusted-life-years," or DALYS, is a measurement of the years of life lost due to the prevalence of a disease. The World Health Organization used DALYS as a metric for allocating scarce development dollars, which helped it to pivot from its historical focus on preventing specific diseases "from above" to building medical infrastructure in local communities for basic care, decreasing sickness "from below." If we return to Sam in the ICU during the pandemic, with George and Brianna in the waiting room, we see that Emanuel's view entails kicking Sam out of the ICU and admitting both 20-year-olds, who will likely live many decades from successful treatment, an option unlikely for an 85-year-old man with many medical problems. In 2010, bioethicist-physician Doug White softened Emanuel's utilitarianism with Kantian elements by not automatically excluding the oldest, most cognitively impaired, or most medically burdened.[16] Instead, he urged maximizing: numbers saved, years gained, and chances of those with the least prospects of living through life's stages. He did criticize maximizing the number of patients who survive to discharge, believing this to be short-sighted.

SAINTS AND SACRIFICE

After the Fukushima nuclear meltdown in 2011, 200 elderly Japanese citizens volunteered to help clean up the plant, arguing that younger workers should not be subject to the dangerous radiation there.[17] Larry Churchill, a 75-year-old bioethicist who retired from Vanderbilt University, similarly wrote that should he become sick with the virus and if Covid patients overwhelmed his local hospitals, he would forgo hospitalization, or being placed on a ventilator, in favor of younger patients who had not lived a full life.[18] Churchill argued along much the same lines as Tennessee bioethicist John Hardwig, whose famous essay "Is there a Duty to Die?" argued that elderly parents cannot expect middle-aged children to become slaves to their late-life care, in the process destroying their own lives.[19] For both bioethicists, not consuming scarce resources as an elderly patient is part of their respect for intergenerational justice. For Churchill, "Part of the moral meaning of aging lies in a sense of reciprocity across generations."[20]

Similarly, devout Jews, Christians, or Muslims might give up their place in the lifeboat for a younger person and be rewarded in the afterlife. In real life, some donate a kidney to strangers. These people are heroes, with saint-like motives, and worthy of emulation. However, and as philosopher J.O. Urmson once wrote, to say they are saints or heroes is also to say that they go beyond the requirements of morality, that in the language of ethics, their actions are *supererogatory.*[21] If ordinary people decline to leave the lifeboat or decline to donate a kidney, they are not bad people. Ordinary morality does not require such sacrifices.

COVID, COGNITIVELY CHALLENGED PATIENTS, AND RIGHTS OF DISABLED PERSONS

Before 2020, several states had established guidelines for distribution of scarce medical resources during a pandemic. New York State had these, over a hundred pages long, but they proved too wordy for practical usage. Alabama and the state of Washington also had such documents, which stated that patients should be excluded from getting ventilators if they had end-stage organ failure and/or, controversially, "intellectual disability or complex neurological problems."[22] When Covid made ventilators scarce in New York, disability advocates who represented children with intellectual disabilities immediately challenged these guidelines in Alabama and Washington, arguing that they would triage their kids, and complained to the Office of Civil Rights of Health and Human Services, alleging violations of the Americans with Disabilities Act. This Office agreed with their complaint and threatened to take Alabama and Washington to federal court. Shortly thereafter, the plans vanished from the websites of Alabama and Washington and state officials there announced that new plans would no longer discriminate against citizens with disabilities.

During this time, bioethicist-physician Joseph Fins, who had previously championed the rights of patients in long-term comas and who helped create the new diagnosis of *minimally conscious states*, helped craft a 2010 report from the New York State Task Force on Life and the Law.[23] This report's guidelines, helped by the late disability advocate Adrienne Asch, used Sequential Organ Failure Assessment (SOFA) scores to prioritize ventilator allocation: Blue—despite maximal efforts, not likely to survive the acute infection; Green—sick but does not need a ventilator; Red—if receives a ventilator, most likely to survive; Yellow—intermediate between Red and Blue. As advocates for people with disabilities, Fins and Asch worried about what they called "crypto discrimination," such as heart conditions associated with Down syndrome, which might mask unjust screening for Down syndrome, even when these conditions had no bearing on survival. The color-coded classification of SOFA avoided such covert discrimination.

Within the medical profession, SOFA is not without its critics. Suppose hospitals must choose between two Covid patients: a previously healthy, 45-year-old high-school teacher and a 75-year-old-man with incipient dementia, and only one can get the ventilator or only one can be admitted to the ICU. Should we really just flip a coin about who we choose? Under the veil of ignorance, wouldn't we want to choose the teacher? Even if we were the 75-year-old man? What if the teacher was a single mother of two children? Isn't care ethics right that being a parent should matter?

During the spring surge in cases in New York City, hospitals and New York officials never used the Task Force's 2010 guidelines, perhaps fearing invoking a triage plan. Instead, hospital administrators forced decisions to trickle down to individual emergency rooms and ICU floors, sometimes with ethics consults.[24]

UNEXPECTED ALLOCATION ISSUES

What experts did not anticipate in the early months of the pandemic was that allocation issues would not only be acute within a hospital—about allocating ventilators, ICU beds, or admission to the hospital—but also system-wide, as was the case at least in northern Italy and in the United States, where huge numbers overwhelmed hospital systems. At first, it was an individual hospital in Italy or the United States that could not handle all the patients, but then as the numbers swelled, it became obvious that it made no sense for a hospital in one part of a state to deny admission to Covid patients while another had open beds. A regional plan was needed.

As the months of the pandemic passed by, another unanticipated issue was the cumulative toll on medical staff. Some nurses spent more hours a day in full protective gear than without, and when they needed a drink of water or had to use the restrooms, they had to completely de-gown. Some emerged from rooms with wet masks and sweat running down their faces, as one said, "all hot and stinky."[25] In New York City during the deluge in March 2020, for some nurses the number of patients needing their intensive care rose from 5 to 10 or even 15, and as ICU beds filled, the only vacancy occurred when a patient died. On some shifts, nurses had to call four families each evening about deaths. The pandemic also hit rural hospitals hard. They often lacked enough nursing staff to handle admitted patients, the numbers of whom set records week after week. A nation-wide pool of nurses moved to hot zones, often for triple pay, but competition soon arose for them. During 2020, the cavalier attitude of those who wouldn't take the virus seriously depressed medical personnel: "I feel like the 20,000 people who died in New York died for nothing," said one, his views echoed by thousands of doctors and nurses as the American death toll soared to half a million, during which "Covid-deniers" still refused to wear masks or to distance themselves.[26]

Unexpected ethical issues emerged in New York City during its surge. Over the eight weeks of the surge, bioethicist Joseph Fins and his team were on call 24/7 supporting nurses, residents, and unit chiefs, providing hundreds of ethics consultations, including questions they'd never previously considered, such as whether to withhold CPR from a dying Covid patient without a signed DNR order (required by New York's laws), or whether to allow a patient sick with Covid to be discharged to a home where he had to live close to others.[27] The original guidelines of New York also did not anticipate ethical problems raised by structural inequities, where poor patients at public hospitals in the Bronx and Queens fared worse than those in Manhattan at private hospitals.

FURTHER READING

Churchill, Larry R. "On Being an Elder in a Pandemic." *Hastings Bioethics Forum*. 13 April 2020.

Emanuel, Ezekiel J., et al. "Fair Allocation of Scarce Medical Resources in the Time of Covid." *New England Journal of Medicine* 382 (21 May 2020): 2049–55.

Fins, Joseph. "Disabusing the Disability Critique of the New York State Task Force Report on Ventilator Allocation." *Hastings Bioethics Forum*. 1 April 2020.

MacIntyre, Alasdair. *A Short History of Ethics*. New York: Macmillan, 1966.

Noddings, Nell. *Caring: A Feminine Approach to Ethics and Moral Education*. Berkeley: University of California Press, 1984.

CHAPTER 6

DEVELOPING VACCINES

Today we take it for granted that vaccines exist to immunize us against dreaded infectious diseases, but this has not always been true. In Daniel Defoe's famous *A Journal of the Plague Year*, an account of the 1665 bubonic plague in London, he wrote,

> The contagion despised all medicine; death raged in every corner; and had it gone on as it did then, a few weeks more would have cleared the town of all, and everything that had a soul. Men everywhere began to despair; every heart failed them for fear; people were made desperate through the anguish of their souls, and the terrors of death sat in the very faces and countenances of the people.

Plague and other pandemics attacked people around the globe for much of human history until scientists discovered remedies, one of them being vaccines.

A BRIEF HISTORY OF VACCINES

In many ways, when Edward Jenner, an English physician and scientist, created the first vaccine for smallpox in 1796, he was both lucky and unethical. Jenner learned that milkmaids infected with cowpox could not be infected with smallpox. He did not understand then, as we do now, the ideas of germ theory or immunity, but he hoped that by deliberately infecting healthy people with the much milder cowpox, he could somehow protect them from smallpox. In an action that would be considered unethical today, he infected eight-year-old James Phipps with pus from a milkmaid who was herself infected with active cowpox. A week later, little James became ill as if he had the flu, but by the second week he had recovered. Six weeks later, Jenner exposed James to live smallpox and fortunately, nothing happened. Little James resisted infection and Jenner became famous, later becoming physician to King George IV of Britain.

This would not be the first time that a physician or scientist became famous and did so while crossing ethical lines.[1] But would Jenner's actions have been considered unethical in 1796? The answer depends on whether one thinks certain ethical rules are timeless, or whether such rules are relative to one's historical era. In 1822 on Mackinac Island, physician William Beaumont treated Alexis St. Martin, a young Canadian fur trader, for a bullet wound to his stomach that left a hole, which Beaumont intentionally left open so he could observe the then-little-understood process of gastric digestion. Beaumont tricked St. Martin into being his man-servant, partly to continue his scientific observations, a relation-ship that made St. Martin mad (he ran away, but Beaumont had him captured and returned). Today several hospitals bear Beaumont's name.

Jenner's discovery explains the origins of the word "vaccine," because *vaca* in Latin means "cow," *vaccinus* means "from cows," and the English "vaccine" means "pertaining to or from cows." One might think that after Jenner's discovery, doctors would immediately try to create other vaccines, but that did not happen. Indeed, it took nearly a hundred years before a French chemist, Louis Pasteur, cre-ated the next vaccine. In 1881, the chicken industry hired Pasteur to cure "chicken cholera," which he did by creating a weakened strain of the chicken-cholera bacte-rium. (The French food-and-beverage industry later hired Pasteur to make wine and milk safe, hence the "Pasteurization" of milk.) By creating weakened, hybrid vaccines, Pasteur cured chickens of cholera and, later, cattle of anthrax, training their immune systems to develop antibodies against real infections.[2]

Pasteur's great challenge came in trying to cure rabies in humans. Rabies today is a preventable, viral disease, and in North America it is still found in wild bats, raccoons, skunks, and foxes. If a rabid animal bites or scratches someone, the person often gets infected. In developing countries today, most rabies deaths worldwide come from feral, rabid dogs. The rabies virus infects the central ner-vous system and the brain, ultimately resulting in death. In Pasteur's time, rabies infections were 100 percent fatal to humans and each year killed a quarter mil-lion people. Fortunately for Pasteur, after a bite, rabies has an incubation period of weeks to months before it attacks a person's brain and kills them.

Microscopes in Pasteur's time could reveal only bacteria, which are much larger than viruses. How small are viruses? To give some idea, almost 55 million Zika viruses could fit on the period at the end of this sentence.[3] As discussed, we know now that viruses make tiny errors in replicating, causing antigenic drift, and when they do, they may interact with viruses in other species, creating hybrid viruses. This happens all the time and is normal in the reproductive life of viruses. Occasionally, hybrid viruses create serious illness in humans, such as swine flu in 2009, SARS1 in Hong Kong in 1997, and SARS2 in 2020.

Just as some hybrid viruses become stronger (and more virulent) to humans, others become weaker. Although he did not know the causative agent, Pasteur nevertheless worked backwards to create a weaker, hybrid version of (what he must have thought of as) "Germ X," to serve as a vaccine for rabies. He infected experimental rabbits with rabid blood from dogs. He then created conditions to weaken Germ X in his rabbits, such as drying the spinal cords of deceased rabbits and extracting from this the dried material of Germ X. Using the same method that worked with chickens and cattle, Pasteur eventually produced a weakened, hybrid version of the rabies virus, gave it to healthy rabbits, exposed them later to real rabies, and voilà!—the healthy rabbits did not get sick.

But what about humans? Could Pasteur use the weakened version of his dog-rabbit-hybrid rabies vaccine on humans? Given that infection by rabies was 100-percent fatal, would it be ethical to inject any human volunteer with experimental vaccines, knowing that some might fail? On July 6, 1885, Pasteur got the opportunity he needed: a rabid dog had bitten nine-year-old Joseph Meister not once but 14 times. Not a physician, Pasteur asked his friend Dr. Grancher to inoculate little Joseph with his weakened dog-rabbit vaccine. Under Pasteur's supervision, Grancher injected Joseph with 13 doses over 10 days. Doses of Pasteur's virus were progressively fresher, more virulent, and stronger, strengthening Joseph's immune system to fight the real rabies virus incubating inside him. Miraculously to his parents and to the world at the time, little Joseph never developed rabies. As it did for Jenner and later Jonas Salk, the world instantly hailed Pasteur as a hero. He had saved an innocent child from certain death and spared humanity from thousands of needless deaths in the future. In the remainder of his life, Pasteur made other major discoveries, and today the Pasteur Institute in France carries on his work.

In the century that followed, scientists used the methods of Jenner and Pasteur to create other vaccines. From live, attenuated, hybrid viruses, they created vaccines for measles, mumps, rubella (aka "German measles" or "three-day measles"), chickenpox, and many forms of influenza.[4] In the 1920s, French researchers used toxins from diseases to make vaccines against diphtheria, tetanus and whooping cough. In the 1930s, American researchers made a vaccine against yellow fever from a version of the virus grown in mice and chickens. In the 1940s, American Thomas Francis grew a flu virus in eggs of chickens and killed it with formaldehyde, for the first time creating a vaccine against flu using a dead virus. (As we will see, it is important that vaccines do not include live virus, even in weakened forms.)

Next came Jonas Salk and his famous cure for polio. As described in Chapter 2, during the 1950s in North America, polio was a dreaded, terrible disease that mysteriously struck down children between ages 5 and 25 and could quickly render them paralyzed for life. Summer outbreaks inexplicably infected tens of thousands of children, leaving hundreds paralyzed and a few dead. Americans and Canadians feared their children getting polio almost as much as they feared the atomic bomb. Some infected children had to live the rest of their lives in iron lungs, a terrible fate for a previously healthy youngster and a tragedy for their family. As was the case in the early days of HIV, no one knew that it was a virus that caused polio and that it spread through contaminated water. Inspired in part by President Franklin D. Roosevelt's personal experience with polio, which caused paralysis below the waist, thousands of US citizens banded together to fund polio research through the newly formed March of Dimes Foundation.

Salk's vaccine worked, but it had two problems. First, he was so sure that it would be effective that he used his own children as guinea pigs, giving it to them first. But his second problem dwarfed this ethical misstep. In April 1955, more than 200,000 children in five American states received a polio vaccine, the world's first effort at mass vaccination. Alas, in the rush to get this vaccine to thousands of children, the process of inactivating the live polio virus proved to be defective. Within days after first vaccinations, reports surfaced of paralysis in vaccinated children; after a month, authorities abandoned the program.

Subsequent investigations revealed that the children had been vaccinated with live polio virus. It was manufactured by the California-based family firm Cutter Laboratories and had caused 64,000 cases of polio, leaving 164 children with varying degrees of crippling, life-long paralysis and killing 10 of them. The heroic, miraculous cure turned into a tragedy. Salk himself was not to blame. In its rush to save children, some critics say that the federal government did not adequately supervise the firms producing the vaccine, while others blamed Cutter Labs. Either way, the rush to create a vaccine became a cautionary tale for Operation Warp Speed, and this "Cutter Incident" started the modern anti-vaccination movement.

As described in Chapter 2, a small number of people receiving the swine flu vaccine in 1976 developed Guillain-Barré Syndrome, and subsequent, successful lawsuits against vaccine companies in the early 1980s caused vaccine shortages and a growing reluctance in parents to give children the standard DPT vaccine (against diphtheria, whooping cough, and tetanus). To counter these legal trends, in 1986 the United States created the National Vaccine Injury Compensation Program, a no-fault alternative to lawsuits in courts, where Special Masters of the US Court of Federal Claims hear cases in a special vaccine court.

The Cutter incident, and others like it, should not make us reject all vaccines, which have brought enormous benefits to humankind.[5] Consider the life of Maurice Hilleman, whose vaccines have saved more lives than any other medical scientist of the twentieth century. Hilleman, an American microbiologist who specialized in vaccinology, developed over 40 vaccines, an unparalleled record of productivity. Of the 14 vaccines routinely recommended in current vaccine schedules, he developed eight, including those for measles, mumps, hepatitis A, hepatitis B, chickenpox, meningitis, pneumonia, and some forms of flu. Because of Hilleman's work, perhaps a billion humans have lived who otherwise might have been killed by infectious diseases—a wonderful epitaph for any scientist, or indeed any human being. An unsung hero, Hilleman is virtually unknown today.

KINDS OF VACCINES

As the history of vaccines above has suggested, different kinds of vaccines exist. First, *whole virus vaccines* use attenuated forms of the whole virus. Historically, this is the most typical vaccine, with examples including vaccines against measles, chickenpox, mumps, and rubella, where vaccines started with live virus and then killed or weakened them because this was the only way to make a vaccine. However, the Cutter Incident showed the danger of using live virus in any way, so scientists searched for other ways to make vaccines.

Second, a new way is to create *viral vector vaccines* that take part of a harmless virus and modify it to look like the virus of a lethal, infectious disease. Virologists use parts of this modified virus to train the immune system to respond to the real virus and, as Pasteur did, to gradually strengthen the system against it. The vaccine for horses against West Nile virus exemplifies this kind.

Third, *mRNA vaccines* constitute a new way to make vaccines and were used in developing the Pfizer and Moderna vaccines for Covid. They avoid using a weakened or deadened germ, and to quote the CDC, "mRNA vaccines...teach our cells how to make a protein—or even just a piece of a protein—that triggers an immune response inside our bodies. That immune response, which produces antibodies, is what protects us from getting infected if the real virus enters our bodies."[6] These vaccines instruct our cells to make a harmless piece of the spike protein that is found on the virus. Once the message is given, the body's cells break down the instructions and eliminate them. The immune system recognizes the harmless spike protein as a substance that doesn't belong there and builds an immune response in the form of antibodies to fight all cells that contain spike proteins, including SARS2. The body thus learns to protect against the spike protein of, in the case of Covid, the coronavirus infection.

These vaccines are not "gene therapy." The vaccines enter muscle cells and express the spike protein. In contrast, gene therapy requires that new material be fully integrated into a host's genes, but the RNA of these vaccines is never integrated in this way. Both the Pfizer and Moderna vaccines contain instructions for replicating the famous spike of the SARS2 virus, making the vaccinated person's immune system think it is being invaded by the real virus, so it produces antibodies against that virus to resist it. The first dose primes the immune system to fight SARS2, and the second builds it up more, so that when the SARS2 really comes along, it can be resisted. Of course, the beauty of these RNA vaccines is that neither uses weakened or dead coronavirus to induce immunity, so neither can mistakenly infect people and cause Covid.

Fourth, *virus-particle vaccines* do just as the name implies. They use particles of the virus that contain pieces of proteins. The advantage of this kind of vaccine, as opposed to whole-virus vaccines, is that they can't cause disease because they don't contain the virus in any form. The vaccine for Human Papilloma Virus (HPV) is an example of this kind.

ETHICAL ISSUES IN DEVELOPING VACCINES

Historically, most experimental vaccines against viruses fail, and they can do so in many ways. Even if they produce *some* antibodies against the virus, antibodies from a vaccine may not produce *enough* antibodies or they may neutralize a virus for only a few months but then fade, requiring an additional booster shot or a new shot every year. Antibodies are protective proteins produced by the immune system to ward off invading germs.

In the United States and most of the developed world, creation of a new vaccine goes through five stages (but only four are named as official phases), like any new drug or device. First, the vaccine is tested in animals. For vaccines intended for humans, that means primates. With the coronavirus, monkeys provided *proof of concept* by showing that some experimental vaccines protected them from getting sick when injected with SARS2.

The first phase with humans is the most dangerous and least understood. Called Phase I by the Food and Drug Administration, its goal is determining if the experimental vaccine is safe in humans. In this phase, researchers look for adverse reactions, either to the vaccine itself or to ingredients used to create it. For this reason, this phase usually involves a small number of people, usually about 40. At this stage, researchers want to test only very healthy people who could withstand unexpected, adverse reactions. Phase I is the level where human subjects are first exposed to experimental risk. Phase I trials are also *open label trials*, where everybody is told they will actually get an experimental vaccine; that is, there are no placebos (see below) in this stage.

The most important, but poorly understood, aspect of Phase I trials is seeing how much of a new drug or vaccine can be given before it harms people. In the typical Phase I trial, dosage is steadily increased until the patients get ill, which is why they are also called *dose-escalation trials*. Obviously, some people will get sick at this stage because the goal is to discover where illness occurs. People have been called heroes for volunteering for Phase I trials of vaccines for Covid, but one wonders if the average volunteer who has given informed consent could pass a multiple-choice quiz on the differences between the three major phases of vaccine/drug trials. Although the consent may be technically "informed," it may not be educated.

Several problems might occur in Phase I. First, the manufacturer might mistakenly use live virus in a vaccine rather than a deadened or weakened version. Second, the volunteer's immune system might overreact and create a cytokine storm, making volunteers seriously ill or even killing them. And third, volunteers might react badly, not to the modified virus or genetic material, but to something used as a substrate for that material, for example, anything from chicken eggs to thimerosal, a preservative containing mercury used in multi-dose flu vaccines, which inhibits the growth of dangerous microbes and which vaccine skeptics dislike.

In Phase I of Moderna's Covid vaccine, three groups of 15 people got different dosages while researchers monitored them to see how they tolerated different dosages. Before Phases II or III began, researchers took serum from inoculated volunteers and examined it to see what antibodies it contained. In Moderna's Phase I, those who received the highest dosage produced the greatest number of good antibodies.[7] What are "good antibodies?" Even to one virus, the body produces many kinds of antibodies, and here researchers sought antibodies that bind to spike proteins on the coronavirus and neutralize it, hence the name *neutralizing antibodies*. In other words, researchers wanted antibodies that prevented the coronavirus from infecting other cells and reproducing.

Elderly patients have diminished immune systems and need stronger dosages than 20-year-olds.[8] So an important ethical question in Phase I, and in developing vaccines in general, is "best dosage for whom?" Unfortunately, research on vaccines often neglects seniors, focusing more on children and on young adults. As a director at the Johns Hopkins Institute for Vaccine Safety said, "We haven't been designing vaccines for the elderly for a long time."[9] Because those over 65 are most at risk for hospitalization and death from Covid, NIH Director Francis Collins quipped, "It would not be particularly encouraging if we have a vaccine that's capable of protecting 20-year-olds who probably have a pretty low risk anyway of getting sick and doesn't work at all for people over 65."[10] That's why we should create several kinds of vaccines and then test each one on different age groups. Already we know that flu vaccines work better on the young than on seniors: some protect up to 90 percent of children but as few as 30 percent of seniors.[11] To get working immunity, seniors might need a booster shot or shots more often.

Once Phase I studies are complete, researchers begin Phase II, calculating the best dosage of the drug or vaccine. Normally this would involve 500 to 800 volunteers, half of whom get a *placebo*, an inert substance with no medical effect. With the Moderna vaccine for Covid, researchers combined Phase I and Phase II, skipping the many months involved in a normal, scaled Phase I study.

Phase III tests each vaccine in 30,000 volunteers, where half get a placebo. Here researchers need varied volunteers, young and old, from all ethnic groups. Phase IV occurs after a vaccine is licensed and when the FDA monitors the creation, distribution, and unintended side-effects of vaccines.[12] So the caretaking role of the government in protecting the health of the nation is not over when it grants manufacturers a license to give vaccines.

Importantly, none of the vaccines against Covid in early 2020 had actually been fully licensed but instead were given "emergency use" authorization, a standard requiring less proof of safety than that for full licensing. These companies must continuously provide data to the FDA's Advisory Committee on Immunization Practices to show that their vaccine continues to be safe for all kinds of people. Indeed, in the technical language of medicine, an "adverse event" from giving a vaccine must legally be reported to the Vaccine Adverse Event Reporting System, or VAERS.[13]

SPEEDING UP DEVELOPMENT OF EXPERIMENTAL VACCINES

When everyone realized the seriousness of the Covid global pandemic, many concluded that vaccines might be the only way to contain the coronavirus. Without them, worldwide deaths from Covid might match those of the Spanish flu. Unfortunately, vaccines typically take years to create and cost millions. Could the process be accelerated?

Some answers quickly emerged. First, do quick studies in primates, followed by quick Phase I studies. Animal studies can be quite long, but were shortened when ACT UP, the HIV-infected activists' group, demanded in 1983 that they be allowed to test the first drug for HIV, AZT (zidovudine). Anthony Fauci agreed, and the drug worked. Second, collapse Phase I and II, or Phase II and III, with large human trials. For the usual 30,000 volunteers, half get a placebo and half get dosages over a range. Afterwards, *lookback studies* determine what dosage worked best. Third, use *human challenge trials* or, simply, challenge trials, which occur when humans volunteer not only to receive an experimental vaccine for a new infectious disease but also to be deliberately infected or "challenged" with that disease to see if the vaccine works. People volunteer this way to help science, to speed up approval, to help humanity, and to get vaccinated against a disease that might affect them.

Without challenge studies, researchers would give experimental vaccine to volunteers in an area with a high incidence of the virus, called a *hot zone*. In 2020, because they had contained the virus, Iceland, New Zealand, and South Korea were not hot zones, but the United States, Brazil, and Russia were; therefore, they were ideal for testing vaccines. Even in hot zones, whether vaccinated subjects get exposed to the virus is random, and testing of vaccines can take a year or longer. Challenge trials avoid any delays. Bioethicist Julian Savulescu of Oxford's

Uehiro Centre for Practical Ethics commented, "I'm surprised they haven't used it earlier. Every day that you delay developing a vaccine and effective treatment, another 5000 people die."[14]

One ethical problem arises in challenge trials: half of the volunteers get a placebo and have no protection against the virus injected into them. Some might have otherwise escaped the virus and never been infected. Is it ethical to infect them and use them as controls for the benefit of humanity?[15] One could reply that if volunteers getting placebos live in hot zones, they likely would have become infected anyway, so even if they get a placebo, get infected, and get sick, they are no worse off than otherwise.

Bioethicists Peter Singer and Richard Yetter Chappell championed human challenge trials for vaccines against Covid.[16] They argued that normal ethical restraints on research, which avoid exposing volunteers to unnecessary risk, do not hold during the abnormal times of pandemics. They claimed that we should allow volunteers to participate in vaccine trials if they give real, informed consent and they volunteer for the greatest good of humanity. The advocacy group One Day Sooner, by early spring 2021, had enlisted over 38,000 volunteers from 166 countries for such trials.[17]

Singer and Chappell invoked the history of smallpox. Recall from Chapter 2 that before Jenner's vaccine, healers in India and Africa used variolation as a crude vaccine because people who received low dosages of infectious viruses became less sick if exposed later to the real virus. Thus, even volunteers who get placebos and who then get exposed to low dosages of SARS2 are likely to experience only mild illness and not full-blown Covid, so the risk to them of serious harm is minimal. Singer and Chappell then argued,

> If we can gain solid evidence that receiving a low dose of the virus leads to a mild case of covid-19, and that such mild cases then bring immunity to further exposure to the virus, we would have found a means of saving hundreds of thousands of lives—and millions of livelihoods. In these circumstances, it seems both reasonable and ethical to invite healthy young volunteers to receive a low dose of the virus, followed by quarantine and medical observation.[18]

They concluded that the longer it takes to understand COVID, "the more lives will be lost." Utilitarianism justifies this conclusion: even if some volunteers are harmed, the good to the world outweighs this harm.

Eventually, 131 bioethicists, philosophers, physicians, and scientists—including Singer, Arthur Caplan, Sally Satel, Daniel Wikler, and 15 Nobel Laureates—signed a letter to NIH director Francis Collins supporting challenge trials.[19] They argued that such trials should be conducted with young, healthy volunteers—not members of vulnerable groups—who when sickened would get the "highest quality medical care" and achieve "robust" informed consent, including "multiple tests of comprehension." Notably, this letter did not specify whether such ideal medical care should be free. However, they did cite altruistic donation of kidneys to strangers, which society already allows.

Another argument arose from Nir Eyal and colleagues at Rutgers University's Center for Population-Level Bioethics,[20] who advocated subjecting healthy volunteers to experimental vaccines, then subjecting them to very low dosages of SARS2, and then comparing them to another group of the same age and health who were naturally infected with SARS2. Instead of arguing from acceptance of living kidney donation as did the 131 signers of the letter above, Eyal et al. argued from our acceptance of doctors and nurses who voluntarily travel to hot zones to treat Covid patients. To minimize risks, these bioethicists advocated recruiting volunteers for challenge studies only from hot zones.

Three dissenting bioethicists doubted whether challenge trials would speed up development because such trials face a trade-off: if we use healthy, young volunteers, then such volunteers may not predict how the vaccine works in unhealthy, senior subjects.[21] If we don't use such vulnerable subjects, then new vaccines could not be ethically distributed to such subjects because the vaccine hadn't been tested on them. As mentioned in Chapter 3, some people ancestrally descended from Africa and Latin America may have a higher genetic susceptibility to serious illness and death from Covid. If they are not substantially represented in challenge trials, then the expected speed-up might not occur. Yet if they are included and get placebos, they are the ones most likely to be hurt by deliberate exposure to SARS2.

As will be discussed in Chapter 11, a continuing issue in research ethics is that African Americans and Latinx citizens in the United States hesitate to volunteer for research. Nevertheless, African Americans and Latinx, who may well be more vulnerable to SARS2 and who urgently need an effective vaccine against it, may be reluctant to participate in human challenge trials. If that is true, then human challenge trials might not be a panacea because they then would not be representative of the populations that most need an effective vaccine.

Now consider a much stronger ethical objection to human challenge trials. The implicit assumption behind most of the arguments discussed so far is that if the vaccine doesn't work, the worst that can happen is that volunteers get sick from Covid in a way that might have happened anyway. But what if that assumption isn't true? What if the vaccine could make volunteers worse-off, or even more likely to die?

Good ethics follows the facts, and there are specific worries about vaccines for coronaviruses. First, a little background. In some coronavirus vaccines, a dangerous immunological phenomenon called *antibody dependent enhancement* occurs. A version of immune enhancement, it is worrisome because in an experimental vaccine for SARS2, it would allow quicker penetration of the coronavirus, making volunteers much sicker than they would have been than if they had contracted the coronavirus naturally.[22] One way in which this could happen is by means of a cytokine storm.

Something like this appears to have happened with Dengvaxia, the only available Dengue fever vaccine, made by a French drug company, Sanofi. A virus carried by mosquitoes causes Dengue fever, which in victims creates fever, joint pains, rashes, and vomiting. In some severe cases, the disease creates dangerous fever, profuse bleeding, hypotension, and systemic shock. Worldwide, it still infects nearly 400 million people and kills 40,000 per year.[23] In the Philippines in 2016, Sanofi vaccinated 830,000 children with Dengvaxia and told their parents that the vaccine would save their kids from getting Dengue fever or from being hospitalized. Four variants of Dengue fever were then circulating in the Philippines, where the virus is endemic, and parents were told that Dengvaxia protected their children against all variants. In truth, the vaccine did protect most children who were previously exposed and who were likely to be exposed again, which was true of most of the 830,000 children who were vaccinated. However, parents were *not* told that for a small percentage of children who by age nine had never been exposed to one of the four variants of Dengue fever, Dengvaxia could make them worse-off.[24]

It appears that Dengvaxia made their immune systems hyper-respond to any variant of viruses causing Dengue fever. Some vaccinated children were hospitalized, and some died, all of which was extensively reported by the Philippine media. Here was a perfect storm of apparent evil, right out of John le Carré's 2001 novel *The Constant Gardener*: a big pharmaceutical company from a rich, Western country testing a dangerous vaccine on innocent children in a developing country, killing some. When Sanofi told the truth to the Philippine public, parents revolted, and all Dengvaxia vaccinations were canceled. Afterwards, because they had not been vaccinated, more children caught Dengue fever. At the very least, researchers should have told all parents the truth and nothing but the truth: that for the benefit of most children, all children would be vaccinated, but some would thereby be worse off or even die.

In extrapolating to challenge studies in adults for vaccines against Covid, we need to ensure that those deliberately vaccinated and infected with mild versions of SARS2 don't later get much sicker when exposed naturally to SARS2, for example, from over-reaction of their immune systems. Presumably, ethical people would want to ensure this before human challenge trials begin. But how can this be guaranteed without performing the trials? Defenders of challenge trials assume we could find a strain of the virus that would make volunteers sick, but not too sick, but that is uncertain. How a virus interacts with any particular person depends on many factors: genetic makeup, prior history, other medical problems, and even how they work and live. We cannot guarantee that volunteers in challenge studies would get only mildly sick.

Recall that Singer and Chappell use utilitarianism to justify challenge trials, and many bioethicists follow them. But what about Kant? According to his categorical imperative—that moral acts are rational and universalizable rules—innocent people should never be exposed to danger to help other people. For Kant, this falls in the category of *Some Things Must Not Be Done*, no matter how much good might be obtained. But what if adults autonomously agree to challenge trials for the good of humanity? Wouldn't Kant approve? Respect their autonomy? Not necessarily. Kant disapproved of using one's body as a means to helping others.[25] Again, Kant thought this to be an ethical line that should not be crossed.

So what happened in trials for vaccines for Covid? In reality, no challenge trials occurred, as least not in the development of vaccines. Why? Partly because of the above ethical concerns, but partly because in the United States and Brazil, so many people quickly became infected that there was no need. In areas with incidence of the virus over 10 percent, researchers could be quite sure that volunteers would be quickly exposed to SARS2. As German critics of such trials noted, by the time human challenge trials were seriously considered, 11 vaccines against SARS2 were already in Phase II clinical trials.[26] However, in February 2021, England approved a challenge trial of up to 90 volunteers aged 18 to 30 to determine the lowest dose of SARS2 that would reliably infect them, and after that, scientists hoped to use similar challenge trials to test the effectiveness of various vaccines against different dosages of SARS2.[27] Whether those later challenge trials occur presumably depends on whether anyone gets seriously harmed in the first one.

OTHER PROBLEMS WITH VACCINE TRIALS

Some vaccine trials have deeper methodological problems. First, consider the general problem in clinical trials of *survivor treatment selection bias*:

> Unlike patients in a randomized, clinical trial, patients in an observational study choose if and when to begin treatment. Patients who live longer have more opportunities to select treatment; those who die earlier may be untreated by default. These facts are the essence of an often overlooked bias, termed "survivor treatment selection bias," which can erroneously lead to the conclusion that an ineffective treatment prolongs survival.[28]

A second problem may also have occurred, namely, *volunteer selection bias*, because those who signed up for the experimental vaccine may have been mostly white, young, and healthy, or have lived in areas with little virus circulating. Effectiveness in the general population is usually less than efficacy in these trials. For example, vaccine trials for Covid probably didn't include many people who were very overweight, had uncontrolled diabetes, major heart problems, or dementia. Also, the Pfizer and Moderna vaccines must be taken weeks apart, and in the real world, some people—for many reasons—take the first dose but not the second. Volunteer selection bias might also have occurred if volunteers hoped that the vaccine would be successful and then acted to limit their exposure to the virus, something not possible for employees of nursing homes and hospitals.

In other words, none of these vaccines were tested on a randomized sample of people; therefore, when any of these experimental vaccines are given in mass vaccination programs, the uptake by people will be less. In a nutshell, vaccines don't stem pandemics; rather, *mass acceptance* of vaccines does. If many citizens refuse vaccinations, vaccines won't work. Finally, for herd immunity to work, 90 percent of citizens may need to be vaccinated or to have been infected.

If all this weren't enough to show that vaccines are not instant panaceas, remember that vaccines vary in how long they protect people and how well they protect those of different ages. A vaccine might wear off after six months and another dose might be needed. A vaccine might protect children and adolescents, but not seniors, or vice versa. Moreover, as we'll see in the next chapter, it's one thing to produce 50,000 doses of a vaccine for clinical trials but quite another to produce 100 million, especially for companies such as Moderna that are new to producing vaccines. The production has many steps and places for many mistakes, and it typically takes many months.[29] These problems quickly became obvious in 2021 when Pfizer paused its factories in Brussels in order to retool for increased production, thus delaying promised first doses in Europe. AstraZeneca failed to deliver its vaccine on time, roiling European countries and the world.

The Pfizer vaccine involved many possible missteps. It had to be stored and transported at minus 94 degrees Fahrenheit; it had to be thawed, and just before it was given; and it had a window of just a few minutes before a shot had to be given. Then those receiving the shots waited 15 minutes to see if they had any adverse reactions. Then they got a certificate reminding them when they got the first shot and when they needed to return for the second. Finally, they downloaded an application on their smartphone to report any symptoms or problems. All that took a lot of time. In Britain, where vaccinations started a few days before they did in the United States, they had hoped to vaccinate thousands a day but actually only vaccinated hundreds a day.[30] They had hoped to vaccinate residents of "care [nursing] homes," but because the vaccine needed special freezers, it shipped to only 50 British hospitals.[31] Early plans to vaccinate everyone in Great Britain over age 50 "within months" seemed naïve.[32] Indeed, the next chapter explores the many, myriad problems that actually arose in rolling out Covid vaccines.

POLITICS AND VACCINES FOR COVID

As SARS2 cases grew in 2020, American scientists worried that corners would be cut in Operation Warp Speed (OWS),[33] that in mid-October President Trump would identify some promising vaccines (a so-called October surprise), claim they were safe because they had been given to a few thousand volunteers, and roll them out before the presidential election on November 3.[34] Those running Trump's campaign for re-election called a vaccine before the election the "Holy Grail" of their efforts.

Because of his financial conflicts of interests, Dr. Moncef Slaoui would never have been appointed head of OWS in normal times. Slaoui, a former Moderna board member, ultimately oversaw a $1-billion grant to Moderna from OWS. He also owned $10 million in stock of GlaxoSmithKline, which got $2.1 billion from OWS. Moreover, neither Dr. Stephen Hahn, Trump's appointed head of the Food and Drug Administration (FDA) nor Dr. Peter Marks, who oversaw vaccine development within the FDA, ruled out emergency approval of a vaccine, which in fact was how all vaccines got approved and distributed.

In other countries, Russia developed a vaccine and gave it to essential workers but published no data in scientific journals, and many Russians declined to take it.[35] With 150 million people, it needed 300 million doses—no easy task. China tested its vaccine in Brazil and got 50-percent prevention of death and disease. Cuba was developing a vaccine, Soberana, which was in Phase III trials in March 2021.

Ultimately, scientists and the public in the United States pushed back against Operation Warp Speed, and Trump's October surprise did not occur.

CHAPTER 7
ALLOCATING VACCINES

The distribution of vaccines during a pandemic makes everyone a bioethicist. Because a successful vaccine is a life-saving good that almost everyone desires, everyone will naturally be interested in the criteria of vaccine distribution. As a result, everyone will also debate the competing goals of distributing vaccines: minimizing deaths versus returning to normal; protecting the most vulnerable versus vaccinating the most quickly; rectifying racial disparities versus protecting medical staff. Other ethical issues involve how to vaccinate skeptical citizens, whether vaccinations should be mandatory, who counts as essential workers, whether vaccine-trial volunteers deserve priority, and how to achieve herd immunity.

This chapter discusses these issues, as well as the tumultuous rollout of Covid vaccines in Europe, the United States, Canada, and the developing world.

SUCCESS WITH QUICK PRODUCTION OF VACCINES

In an extraordinary development in 2020, under Operation Warp Speed, the Trump administration paid $12 billion for vaccine production and ownership of six experimental vaccines to Moderna, Pfizer/BioNTech, Sanofi, and Glaxo-SmithKline. Neither Moderna nor BioNTech had ever produced a vaccine, and both used new RNA technology. Skeptics doubted if Operation Warp Speed could hurriedly create safe vaccines. The Monday after the presidential election, Pfizer announced that the 44,000 volunteers who received its experimental vaccine had 95-percent protection against getting Covid, defined as getting sick with self-reported symptoms. Only 170 people reported being sick, 162 in the placebo group and only 8 in the vaccine group. For seniors with weaker immune systems, it also reported 94-percent protection.[1]

A vaccine's *efficacy* differs from its *effectiveness*, the latter of which measures how it works in the general population.[2] Pfizer's measure of efficacy depended on volunteers answering truthfully on a smartphone about being sick. A few days later, Moderna reported similar results, and fortunately, its vaccine did not need to be stored at minus 94 degrees. Moderna recruited 7,000 Americans over age 65, 5,000 of whom had heart conditions, diabetes, and/or obesity; a third of volunteers came from communities of color. Even better, in March 2021 the FDA approved Johnson & Johnson's one-shot vaccine, which needed only normal refrigeration.

Importantly, some vaccines are designed to protect against the sickness (in this case, Covid) caused by a virus, while others are designed to protect against infiltration of the body by a virus (in this case, the presence of SARS2). In other words, some vaccines in trials may prevent SARS2 from becoming Covid, while others may block infection of the virus in the first place and give what immunologists call *sterilizing immunity*, which is complete absence of the virus in a person or population. The figures from Pfizer showed that its vaccine protected volunteers against getting sick, against getting Covid, but not from infection by the virus. A vaccine that protected against both would be ideal. Because neither Pfizer nor Moderna tested volunteers for SARS2 when they checked in, they didn't prove that those vaccinated couldn't spread the virus—an important fact for post-vaccination behavior and so-called immunity passports. Preliminary data from the Moderna vaccine did show that three months after the second dose, two-thirds of volunteers neither got sick nor had the virus. Presumably, the other third, who also didn't get sick, may have shown evidence of having the virus.

A week after these announcements, AstraZeneca announced promising, but confusing, results. Because AstraZeneca combined Phase II and III in trials, it got confusing results about the ideal dosage. Paradoxically, a half dosage of its vaccine produced better results than a full dosage. The AstraZeneca vaccine had 76% efficacy for 3 months after just one shot and was easy to store, transport, and administer. It was also cheap because AstraZeneca was providing it at cost. Unfortunately, its rollout had many problems. The FDA did not think it gave adequate proof of its safety, so it did not issue it Emergency Use Authorization.

As noted, Pfizer and Moderna received Emergency Use Authorization for their new vaccines, something the FDA had never authorized before. Given the pandemic's devastation in the United States in mid-December 2020, when deaths had topped 300,000, the FDA understandably authorized both, but everyone quickly seemed to forget that the vaccines were not fully licensed (an important fact for mandatory vaccination). Full licensing requires at least a year of careful follow-up.

England began vaccinating first, and on December 8, 2020, when it vaccinated Margaret Keenan, aged 90, followed by William Shakespeare (yes, that was his real name), aged 81. Some doses of Pfizer's vaccine shipped on December 13, and within days, English hospital personnel got the first shot of the two-shot vaccine. The next day, after 460,000 cases and 13,400 deaths in Canada, a Canadian got the Pfizer vaccine.[3]

Almost immediately, problems of scaling up and delivery emerged: Pfizer could not deliver as many doses as it had promised. Also, despite bragging about using the military to deliver the vaccines within 24 hours, President Trump had never issued the order to do so, and Americans had to rely on UPS and FedEx. This was just the beginning of a colossal failure of distribution, not just in the United States but almost everywhere, as countries tried to plan for how the vaccines would get into people's arms. Even if Pfizer had delivered 20 million doses, enough to give 10 million Americans two doses each, that still left 320 million unvaccinated Americans, as well as 38 million Canadians next door, as well as 130 million in next-door Mexico, all of whom needed two doses of a vaccine that required storage at very low temperatures. For 300 million Americans, the two companies that had never produced vaccines on this scale had a monumental task ahead, one equivalent to the Manhattan Project.[4] Russia confronted the same problem: it had promised St. Petersburg 5 million doses but actually delivered only 30,000.[5]

As one expert commented, "Vaccine manufacturing is an endeavor where an almost infinite combination of things must work perfectly," where variability exists in raw materials, the microorganisms needed to grow key ingredients, the conditions of the cultures in which those microorganisms are grown altogether, "a science with established principles, but sometimes is more idiosyncratic than art."[6] Even so, pressures in 2021 mounted to cut the time of production at Pfizer plants from 100 to 60 days.

THE CDC AND THE STATES

Unlike some countries, the United States had no central authority to allocate vaccines. Although a committee at its Centers for Disease Control issued guidelines (which its CDC director did not need to accept), each state's public health department decided whether to follow these guidelines or devise its own plan. Lack of a national plan to distribute vaccines was a moral failure. Given that every country had many months to devise such a strategy, it was a tragedy that for many of them no plan existed. As the incoming Biden team complained about the distribution plan of the Trump administration, "There was no plan." This resulted in what *USA Today* called, "50 States, 50 Plans."[7] Here is one example:

some states chose not to vaccinate prisoners until all healthy residents were vaccinated, but other states prioritized prisoners before essential workers.

Both the United States and Canada are populated with large numbers of citizens in urban centers on both coasts and around the lower Midwest, with huge rural areas in between. Governors of rural states and provinces allocated vaccines differently from those in urban areas, especially if they had workers vital to their area or political pressures to give vaccines to particular groups. On another front, employers such as Boeing, GM, and Toyota, with thousands of workers, vied to get their employees vaccinated early.

Canada, which secured a huge supply of vaccines and did so early, struggled to move its vaccines from industrial freezers into the arms of Canadians—especially those of long-term care residents. Its decentralized health system, run by individual provinces and territories, didn't help. As in the United States, while the Canadian federal government procured the vaccines and distributed them to its 13 provinces and territories, provincial and territorial officials there decided which groups to prioritize and how to deliver the doses.[8] Provinces with citizens living across large geographical areas had difficulties vaccinating people in their remote, isolated communities.

Because all administrators, as well as every vaccine-distribution committee, had the media, politicians, and impatient citizens looking over their shoulders and second-guessing their decisions, much confusion erupted, and controversy ratcheted through the whole process in both Canada and the United States.

ABILITY TO PAY AND ACCESS TO VACCINES

During pandemics, societies need as many citizens as possible to get vaccinated and to do so as quickly as possible, so vaccines should ideally be provided free. For that reason, in most developed countries, almost everyone vaccinates without charge. Despite a vaccine's effectiveness and the wisdom of making it free to achieve herd immunity, poor countries such as Niger, Yemen, and Haiti may not be able to afford many vaccines. The Pfizer vaccine costs $39 for two doses, which is too much. This makes the $3 AstraZeneca vaccine the only possibility there. For two-shot vaccines, Egypt will charge $12, about a week's wages for a third of its workers. Such a charge will slow herd immunity there.

It is also worrisome that providers may be able to charge for giving vaccines. This happens with donated blood, where the American Red Cross cannot charge for blood but does charge substantial fees for blood typing, storage, and transportation of blood to hospitals.[9] Some news releases indicated that American physicians and pharmacies would charge for giving vaccines. Although fees would incentivize pharmacies and medical clinics to give vaccines, they would also incentivize providers to avoid areas with few people. Also, and this is an insight from behavioral economics, we know that some people, if they had to pay any sort of fee, would refuse vaccination. A marketing study by students in Birmingham, Alabama, once discovered that some insured patients would choose one hospital over another for cardiac bypass surgery (for which the hospital might charge $100,000) because of free valet parking at one hospital that the other lacked. Soon thereafter, almost all hospitals offering such surgery began to offer many free services to such patients.

ALLOCATION PRIORITIES

Allocation Criteria Become News, Not for Ventilators but for Vaccines
Outside bioethics classes, few people knew of the 1962 God Committee, and although educated people had read about agonizing allocation decisions in New York City, most thought those issues to be far removed, but then the new vaccines in 2021 changed everything, and everyone wanted to get vaccinated. Suddenly, newspapers, television networks, and Internet blogs discussed allocation standards, and some groups objected to being left out. What had seemed in 2020 like an issue affecting few people by 2021 had become an ethical issue of global concern.

In Chapter 5, I discussed allocation issues concerning ventilators, but distributing vaccines raised the same issues, only in a new context, and in bioethics, context is everything. For example, taking a 90-year-old patient off a ventilator in favor of a 45-year-old clearly could be a matter of life and death for both, and it's equally clear how using the criterion of maximizing life-years favored selecting the 45-year-old. But the opposite is true for priority for vaccines, because the 45-year-old might have a good chance of surviving infection without a vaccine, but the 90-year-old might not.

Another important fact about context is that the 45-year-old who might get a ventilator if competing with a 90-year-old (because of more life-years gained) might, with a vaccination, easily wait on getting a shot and not be at risk of death from infection, a luxury that 90-year-olds could not afford. Finally, given the lower immune response of 90-year-olds, the vaccines might not work as well in them as in 45-year-olds, or might be more dangerous for them to get. Again, context matters in bioethics.

Who Should Get Vaccines First?
As soon as vaccines arrived, the easiest philosophical job quickly got accomplished: deciding who to vaccinate first. Everyone agreed that front-line medical workers, putting their lives on the line and frequently exposed to SARS2, deserved to be vaccinated first. Most states followed Harvard's Mass General Hospital, giving vaccines first to workers with the most exposure to Covid patients.[10] Various systems did the same, prioritizing workers by risk—either from SARS2 or death from Covid, or both.[11] The CDC placed such workers in what it called "Group 1a."

The ethical questions were not solely about what kind of worker got vaccinated first but also concerned which hospitals and which medical systems got supplies. When one system of hospitals in Atlanta, Maryland, or Texas got vaccines the first week, and other systems got none, those left out quickly complained and did so publicly.[12]

Who Comes Next?

Giving front-line workers priority in access to vaccines acknowledged (a) that they deserved protection for risking their health and life caring for Covid patients; (b) that if they were unvaccinated, they would risk being super-spreaders in their hospitals; and (c) that the greatest long-term good for the greatest number was to keep medical workers healthy and medical systems functioning. This last goal became increasingly important in 2021 as hospitals became overwhelmed with Covid patients, exhausting medical staff in some communities where staff had been treating Covid patients for a year (according to award-winning research by Kaiser Health News, over 3,000 medical workers died in 2020 taking care of patients).[13]

Most bioethicists agreed that those in nursing homes (Group 1b) should come next. Giving the vaccine to those in nursing homes recognized their high Covid mortality rate, which in 2020 was 40 percent nationally in the United States, 70 percent in Connecticut alone, and in December 2020 across the country, averaging 5,000 deaths per week.[14] Canada's long-term care homes were as bad or worse. Giving vaccines to nursing-home patients recognized the standards both of protecting *vulnerable people* and of *avoiding the most deaths*.

In many ways, the easy part was choosing whom to place in Groups 1a and 1b. Yes, give it to millions of medical workers on the front lines and to those in nursing homes, but how do we decide who comes next? Would the next 100 million Americans or Canadians include those with two or more chronic health conditions, those over the age of 65, or those classified in some way as essential? As medical staff began getting vaccines, almost immediately, unions and various industries, from hotel workers to grocery clerks to teachers to Uber drivers, clamored to get the vaccine next.[15] There was no sense among them of "We're all in this together and let's be patient," but rather, "We want ours first and to heck with everybody else." At this point, mass confusion erupted. Every policy guru had an idea about who should go next. Magazines and newspapers filled with columns urging that various groups be vaccinated next. Different states made different decisions. When it comes to vulnerability of at-risk populations, the obvious targets are poor people in homeless shelters, migrant workers living in crowded conditions in cheap apartments or trailer parks, and prisoners. Targeting such groups means that middle-class people would come behind them, an option not popular with politicians.

Everyone had an idea. Former FDA Commissioner Scott Gottlieb agreed with giving the first batches to front-line medical workers and those in nursing homes. He then urged giving the next batch to seniors over age 65.[16] This would be easy to do because anyone in the United States over 65 would be easy to identify, for example with a driver's license. Paul Peterson, a Harvard professor of government and fellow at the Hoover Institution, agreed, arguing that the fastest, most efficient way was to vaccinate anyone over age 65 and not worry about their occupations or risk-factors.[17] Thomas Frieden, former director of the CDC, argued that super-spreaders should be vaccinated in Group 1b, although he was vague about how to identify them or how they would be encouraged to be vaccinated, as well as whether being so identified might harm some people ("My hair stylist was vaccinated as a super-spreader: should I get tested today?").[18]

If the goal is to reduce mortality, we should first vaccinate three groups: medical workers, seniors over age 75, and seniors over 60 with major medical problems. As 90 percent of deaths from Covid occur in people in these groups, about 20 percent of the population, vaccinating them would rapidly decrease mortality from SARS2.[19] Florida decided to simply vaccinate anyone over 65, but some seniors over 65 were from Canada and Argentina, or north Americans only there for the winter. When Florida's vaccines ran out and when Floridians saw out-of-state "snowbirds" getting vaccinated ahead of them, they became angry.

At the same time, two economists argued that after 18 million health-care workers got the vaccine, the nation's 3.3 million teachers should come next.[20] Why? Because doing so was necessary to fully re-open schools, and without such open schools, too many parents couldn't successfully work. Although they didn't explicitly state it, their underlying criterion for distribution was *to get life back to normal* (returning parents to jobs and children to their education).

Race also became involved. Meharry Medical College, an historically Black medical school, implied racist motives when it was snubbed in the first rollout of the Pfizer vaccines (Tennessee's health commissioner replied that she earmarked the first round of Pfizer doses for larger health-care providers because Pfizer only shipped its vaccine in huge batches or "trays").[21] One problem with vaccines such as the Pfizer vaccine was the need for speed and the need to avoid wasting it. Once the vaccine was thawed and mixed with saline solution, nurses had only six hours to use it before it went bad. So it was easiest to first give it to large numbers in cities with big freezers for storing the Pfizer vaccine.

The logistics of vaccinating residents of long-term care or nursing homes in rural areas mounted. CVS and Walgreens each made over 9,000 visits to such homes in the first weeks of 2021, but each home—which averaged 100 residents each—required three visits, the first two to give doses and the third as a backup for residents or staff who had missed a dose.[22] For many, the question of who came next boiled down to who was truly "an essential worker," our next topic.

Who Are Essential Workers?

If we say that the first supply of vaccines should be provided to essential workers, we must then ask, "Essential for *what*?" For driving ambulances and rescuing people? For keeping meat on the table? For keeping kids safe in daycare? For keeping dead bodies from rotting? From keeping us safe from invasion by foreign countries? For restoring power after storms? For picking up garbage? For keeping Internet and cable lines operating? For selling food in grocery stores? Are K–12 teachers essential workers? What about journalists and newspaper delivery personnel? Are professional athletes essential workers for the nation's mental health?

To understand problems of defining essential workers, consider that in the United States, health care includes 6 million workers (physicians, nurses, nursing assistants, licensed and vocational nurses, and medical assistants); law enforcement includes 2 million workers (security guards, patrol officers, and firefighters); cleaning services includes 2 million (janitors and cleaners; housekeepers).[23] Millions of workers in other categories include cashiers, fast-food workers, postal carriers, construction workers, truck drivers, bus drivers, K–12 teachers, workers in meat-processing plants, field workers in agriculture, and delivery workers for the postal service, UPS, FedEx, and Amazon. One institute classified more than 55 million American workers as essential; another classified their number at 74 million.[24]

Because there was no national plan or coordination, each state decided who was an essential worker and in what order they would get vaccinated. Governors of each American state decided which workers were essential. "You could be an essential worker in New York but not in Texas, so all this contributes to the chaos and confusion that employers are having to deal with," said Nadina Rosier, who advises businesses on medical issues affecting workers. The governor of Kansas said that workers in meat-packing plants would be vaccinated next. Delta Airlines asked that its flight attendants get vaccinated early as "front-line workers, but as an international company it had no state Governors to implore."[25]

One problem that arose concerned those workers who would get vaccinated last; would they feel disenfranchised or devalued? On the other hand, wasn't it unavoidable that any priority list would have some workers getting it before others and, thus, some workers feeling undervalued? One solution would be to create transparent, evidence-based, rational criteria in each state about which workers got vaccinated first, and why.

Other Candidates for Early Vaccination

Another criterion for early vaccination was that members of Group 1c should be those with several major medical problems, such as diabetes, alcoholism, or high blood pressure. However, unless all vaccines were given in doctor's offices or hospitals, which seems unlikely, employees would need to reveal such conditions to get vaccinated and, in the process, reveal such hitherto-unknown conditions to employers, which would violate their rights to privacy of medical information.

Saving the most vulnerable is also a plausible criterion for deciding whom to vaccinate early, but it was controversial. Rawlsians would certainly advocate for the most vulnerable, which would include not only residents of nursing homes but also prisoners, those in detention centers for immigrants, and those in homeless shelters. None of these groups had many options for physical distancing, with detained people having the fewest. Indeed, vaccinating prisoners, who are four times more likely to become infected than average citizens, before ordinary Americans, proved especially controversial. Jared Polis, governor of Colorado, said, "There's no way it's [the vaccine] going to go to prisoners before it goes to people who haven't committed any crime."[26] In so deciding, he undermined the plan that Colorado had submitted to the CDC. In Oklahoma, the governor assigned prisoners and their guards, as well as those living in homeless shelters or working in meat-processing plants, to a low listing in the distribution plan.[27] Its plan de-emphasized workers and guards as spreaders of infection in their local communities and prioritized Oklahomans over age 65 or those working in high-density manufacturing plants.[28] In Minnesota, no one was happy with the first allocations, where the famous Mayo Clinic got enough for only 6 percent of its workers and "safety net clinics" seeing high numbers of Covid infections got none. One clinic's leader complained of the state's "trickle down" allocation plan and said it perpetuated historical inequities in Minnesota.[29]

Even if we focus on the most vulnerable, there is an underlying philosophical question, "Vulnerable to what?" To mere exposure? To getting sick with Covid? To dying from Covid? To spreading infection to relatives? Filipino nurses working in the United States comprise 4 percent of nurses but account for 33 percent of Covid deaths among nurses. Do they count as "the most vulnerable"?[30] What about garbage collectors and workers who clean sewage and septic tanks? Because scientists monitor sewage for the incidence of SARS2 on some campuses, we know the virus can be found in sewage.[31] These workers are more vulnerable than tens of millions of professionals who work from home selling insurance, creating ads, or reading fMRI scans.

Should Vaccine Trial Volunteers Who Got Placebos Get Priority?

Volunteers in England, the United States, Brazil, and other countries signed up for vaccine trials, but half got placebos. After the Pfizer and Moderna vaccines were approved, some volunteers who received placebos wanted priority for getting successful vaccines. However, epidemiologists opposed them because long-term data were needed, not just for FDA authorization for emergency use but also for full approval and a license, and because they needed not months but years to prove vaccines that worked well and had few side-effects.

In October 2020, Judith Munz of Phoenix volunteered for a vaccine trial by Johnson & Johnson and then hoped she would get a successful vaccine earlier than otherwise, but she concluded that she only got a placebo. When the Pfizer vaccine launched that December, Judith was denied that vaccine because data from her Johnson & Johnson trial were still needed for two more years.[32] It certainly seems unfair that Judith would be penalized in her attempt at getting a successful vaccine because she had volunteered in a trial for a different vaccine. Anthony Fauci, who is married to bioethicist Christine Grady (head of the Department of Bioethics at the National Institutes of Health Clinical Center), proposed an innovative solution: bring volunteers back and give them a second dosage, where those who got a placebo get the real vaccine and those who got the vaccine get a placebo, with no volunteer knowing who got what.[33] In that way, Fauci said, researchers could still follow both groups over the next years and see if a particular vaccine's protection faded.

A working group at the WHO objected to any strategy that reduced the gold standard of long-term studies of placebo-controlled vaccine trials. With the lives of hundreds of millions of people at stake, it argued that allowing volunteers to test themselves for antibodies (to see if they got a placebo) and then to jump ship to get another vaccine, would hurt the power of the results.[34] These authors, perhaps naïvely, hoped that those who volunteered in vaccine trials "for altruistic reasons would probably understand the value of gathering data" from long-term results and of not unblinding treatment/placebo assignments. All of which raises the question again of whether those volunteering to test experimental vaccines against Covid really understood what they were undertaking.

A Lottery?

Given competing ethical theories of just distribution and competing interests of different groups, not everybody will agree on any allocation scheme; inevitably some group will not be as high on the list as it desires to be. The best that can be done is to balance as fairly as possible many different interests and to be as transparent as possible about the rationales used to make allocation decisions. At some point, reasonable people understand what Aristotle meant when he introduced his *Nicomachean Ethics*: "our account of this science [of ethics] will be adequate if it achieves such clarity as the subject-matter allows; for the same degree of precision is not to be expected in all discussions, any more than in all products of handicraft."[35] Along those lines, a degree of arbitrariness will inevitably be part of any list of prioritized workers for vaccines.

After front-line workers were vaccinated, some bioethicists proposed using *a weighted lottery* for distributing any remaining shots of scarce vaccines. The beauty of a weighted lottery is that although members of some groups might get favorable weights, from the beginning no vaccines are reserved for them. Whoever is weighted more heavily gets their name on the most balls in descending number, until the last person who gets just one ball. Weighted lotteries have been used to select students for elite schools in cities where students from disadvantaged backgrounds are given heavier weights. Weighted lotteries give certain groups better chances of getting vaccines, but chance still governs which particular person gets the vaccine.

Doug White, a bioethicist and critical care physician at the University of Pittsburgh, used a weighted lottery when only one in four patients who needed the drug Remdesivir could actually receive it.[36] When a vaccine or drug is scarce, a hospital needs a rational, transparent way to distribute it. In White's system, a committee of doctors, nurses, and bioethicists ranks patients, deciding which groups should be given preference and how much. First-responders might be more heavily weighted than patients who are unlikely to recover. Those with more life-years to live could be weighted more than those with few years to live. Ashish Jha, the Dean of Public Health at Brown University, and Robert Wachter, chair of the Department of Medicine at the University of California at San Francisco, came to the same conclusion about using a lottery, arguing that after giving vaccines to anyone over age 55, a group of about 97 million Americans, the remaining 150 million Americans should get their vaccines by lottery.[37]

The nice aspect of a lottery is that it is one of the distribution schemes most acceptable to patients. Rather than telling them that they weren't a member of the right ethnic group, or that their job wasn't essential, it's easier to say that their number didn't come up. White says his patients accepted that system: "I speculate that is because we are very transparent about the reason and the ethical framework that applies to everyone who comes into hospital, whether that is the hospital president or someone who is homeless."[38]

As a side point, because allocation within a group is random, weighted lotteries may allow researchers to discover which kind of patients do best on a particular vaccine. For this reason, data from weighted lotteries may be as revealing as those from randomized clinical trials.

A Note on Prioritization

Overall, it may be a mistake to focus too much on who gets vaccinated first and why. Although this may be a strange point to make in a bioethics text, if we focus too much on being fair—focus too much on insuring that the wrong people don't get vaccinated first—we may slow things down so much that the virus wins. There is an old proverb, "The perfect is the enemy of the good," and a perfectly fair system will be a very slow system. Florida may have done a good thing by simply vaccinating everyone—native or not—over age 65 because, after all, snowbirds in Florida can transmit the virus and occupy hospital beds there just as easily as native Floridians.

VACCINATION COMPLEXITIES

Unprofessional Behavior

Politicians did a poor job teaching their citizens patience. The Trump administration, wanting to win an election and take credit for creating vaccines, established unrealistic expectations for quick access to vaccines. When quick access didn't materialize and vaccine scarcity became apparent, many health-care workers, perceiving vaccination as a life-or-death issue, behaved like Titanic passengers, jumping the queue to secure a lifeboat seat. In hospitals that provided vaccines to medical staff directly involved with Covid patients, some lied by saying they were front-line workers.

At Stanford Medical Center, where the Pfizer vaccines were given, only seven of Stanford's 1,500 medical residents—many of whom were taking care of Covid patients—got the vaccine first, and this was from a batch of 5,000 doses.[39] Barnes Hospital in St. Louis adopted a seniors-first policy that bypassed younger, front-line nurses and doctors, who became angry when they had to wait a month for the vaccine.[40] When a marketing staffer at Mount Sinai Hospital in New York City posted pictures of himself on social media getting vaccinated, unvaccinated physicians and nurses fumed at the hospital who cared for Covid patients.[41] At other hospitals, fellow workers outed line-breakers and front-line imposters, irritated at such selfish behavior. Governor Cuomo threatened hospitals and medical practices with fines and revocation of licenses for breaking the rules.[42]

Like the staffer at Mount Sinai, most people who were vaccinated posted a picture on social media, which let everyone know who got vaccinated first. For some, such postings said, "I'm special. You're not," infuriating front-line physicians.[43] In these cases, administrators accustomed to private, internal decisions with no public accountability suddenly saw their decisions revealed on national news, for which they were little prepared. In most cases, they quickly backed down and changed the priorities. Outside medicine, some wealthy people in Palm Beach and New York City tried to game the system to get vaccinated early, sometimes successfully.[44] Such bad behavior slowed down the roll-out, as those in charge sought to verify the status of members of each group, often a time-consuming process.

Volunteering Not to Be Vaccinated?

In Chapter 5, I mentioned bioethicist Larry Churchill, who argued that seniors like him who have had good lives should not access scarce medical resources that might benefit younger people. In a letter to the *New York Times*, 93-year-old Lois Taylor wrote that after fracturing her hip, she had recently spent time in a nursing home, and her visit there convinced her that "some of the residents there may have welcomed an end to their lives."[45] Lois wanted to give her vaccine to those who "have young families and have much to live for." Should we accept Lois's request? Probably not. Lois is thinking about the vaccine only as a possible good to herself, but because she lived in a nursing home with many other frail seniors, taking the vaccine might protect others.

So, yes, if you're living as a senior hermit in a remote part of western Colorado and want to go to the end of the line to let others be vaccinated, go for it! But if you're a senior working checkout at a grocery store, take the vaccine. Don't be a super-spreader.

Dividing Scarce Two-Dose Vaccines?

Several scholars advocated giving one dose of Pfizer's or Moderna's limited vaccines to twice as many people, giving everyone some immunity and later, only after a second dose arrived, reinforcing that dosage.[46] Another posited giving Americans a half dose of the Moderna vaccine twice in order to stretch supplies.[47] The head of Canada's vaccine program, a retired general, suggested giving the two-shot Moderna vaccine as one shot.[48]

In 2021, Great Britain decided to give as many people as possible the first dose of the Pfizer or Moderna vaccines, giving twice as many people some protection. The country delayed the second dose by as much as three months, and if someone couldn't remember which vaccine they got, or if a second dose was unavailable, citizens could get shots of two different vaccines.[49] It accepted the premise that giving twice as many people *good* immunity was better than giving half that number *maximal* immunity. Some British virologists disagreed, fearing that single doses could create vaccine-resistant strains. Others worried that single doses wouldn't prime the immune system enough, and if single-dose vaccinated people later became infected, they might be worse-off.[50] Nevertheless, Britain's gamble appeared to have paid off, getting the country ahead of both the United States and Europe in vaccinating the most of its citizens. Moreover, because vaccinations slow the spread of viruses, Britain seems to have avoided festering problems with the B117 variant that hobbled Europe.

It might seem that utilitarianism would dictate giving twice as many people the first dose of a two-dose vaccine to both protect them and fight the spread of the virus, but that may be more politics than fact. Most scientists wanted to give the vaccine in the way it had been tested in clinical trials, and no other way. The first dose trains the immune system to recognize the virus by injecting harmless versions of some of the coronavirus's key features; the second dose, after the body has been creating antibodies to the coronavirus, jumpstarts the production of those antibodies.[51] Given these facts, it doesn't seem that simply giving the first dose, although it might protect against immediate death and illness for a few weeks after injection, would create long-lasting immunity. A spokesman for Pfizer agreed: "There is no data to demonstrate that protection after the first dose is sustained after 21 days," which is a knock-down argument against giving twice as many people only one dose.[52]

Anthony Fauci added his perspective on the issue:

There really are no data on what happens if you delay the second dose by three months or four months or two months. We don't have any idea what the level of protection is and what the durability of protection is. It's fraught with some danger when you're making a decision about the regimen you're going to use when you don't really have a considerable amount of data. We're holding in reserve that second dose, because we believe we need to go according to what the FDA said is the safe and effective way to use these vaccines.[53]

Moreover, the longer the gap between the first and second doses, the easier it would be to lose track of people who got one dose but not the second. Also, the longer the gap, the more things that can happen to prevent the first-dosers from getting the second shot. Furthermore, any departure from standard protocols would increase distrust about the vaccines. Some people might object to getting only a half or one dose, seeing it as discrimination. Allowing vaccines to be mixed, with different vaccines for the first and second doses, even if both were RNA vaccines, seems especially problematic.

Proponents of giving only one dose of Pfizer got a boost when Israel announced preliminary data, not peer-reviewed, that one dose of Pfizer gave 85-percent immunity against Covid and hospitalization two to four weeks after being given.[54] Pfizer declined to comment, citing incomplete data. Moreover, in one preliminary study, people who recovered from Covid and who got one dose of Pfizer did better than those receiving two doses, and in another study, one dose of Pfizer for UK health workers reduced hospitalizations and deaths by 85 percent, 15 to 28 days after the first dose.[55] Based on these data, some suggested giving elderly and medical workers two doses but everyone else at first only one dose.

Giving only one dose also has big implications for vaccine certificates or immunity passports (see Chapter 10). If the duration of immune response can't be determined for just one dose, the value of such certificates would be undermined. Because the mRNA molecule rapidly degrades (which is why it needs to be stored at freezing temperatures), immunity is likely to degrade three weeks after one shot, which is why a second shot is necessary to remind the immune system of a threat.

In sum, not giving a second dose, giving only a half dose, and allowing people to mix doses of two different vaccines all seem like spur-of-the moment, panicked reactions to problems of accelerating vaccinations. All these attempts inject politics into what should be a purely scientific decision. On the other hand, merely delaying the second dose for a month or two in order to vaccinate twice as many people might be a good strategy for some countries with minimal supplies of vaccines. Along scientific lines, the best solution would be to start randomized clinical trials of delaying the second shot versus administering two shots at intervals, and accessing long-term immunity in both groups.

Allergic Reactions

As explained in Chapter 6, RNA vaccines aren't grown in eggs or cells and don't need to be weakened, killed, or purified in the same way that traditional vaccines do, so we wouldn't expect them to create the severe allergic reactions created by traditional vaccines. At least that was the theory. Because no RNA vaccine had ever been used before in a mass vaccination program, this was not proven, and as it turned out, some people did have allergic reactions to both vaccines. Skeptics suspected that vaccines had been developed too quickly by Operation Warp Speed and might have flaws. Usually, the FDA waits three months for side-effects to appear, but in 2020, it shortened its observational period to two months.[56] Nor were any of the vaccines given normal approval, just "emergency use" approval. To some, that implied a lower standard of safety.

What would such a lower standard involve? The answer depends on what both scientists and informed citizens consider an acceptable percentage of severe allergic reactions. To understand the issue, let's first no longer use the euphemism "side-effect" (although "side-effects" can include death) but focus on *severe reactions* such as anaphylactic shock, a life-threatening overreaction of the immune system. On the first day the Pfizer vaccine was given in Alaska, a nurse who got the shot there went into such shock, needing to be rushed to the emergency room. In Boston, the Moderna vaccine gave a physician a similar reaction.[57] It is possible that their immune systems were already super-charged against polyethylene glycol (PEG), an ingredient in the Pfizer and Moderna vaccines, which had never been used in a vaccine before but which has previously triggered anaphylaxis in some people taking drugs with it. According to a piece in *Science* magazine, "Some allergists and immunologists believe a small number of people previously exposed to PEG may have high levels of antibodies against PEG, putting them at risk of an anaphylactic reaction to the vaccine."[58]

After 5.3 million Americans received the Pfizer or Moderna vaccines, at least 29 experienced an anaphylactic reaction.[59] A 56-year-old physician in Miami with no known medical problems died 16 days after taking the Pfizer vaccine.[60] Four times as many women reported allergic reactions to Covid vaccines as men, according to a CDC study in 2021. The Pfizer vaccine has a rate of severe allergic reactions of 5.5 cases in a million, worse than the rate of the same reactions with most flu vaccines (1.3 cases per million).[61] Of equal importance is the rate of "Grade 3 adverse events," those severe enough to prevent the activities of daily life, including fatigue and muscle pain. Nearly one in five volunteers for the Moderna vaccine aged 18 to 64 had such a Grade 3 reaction, or 17.4 percent of volunteers, a rate much higher than for most vaccines.[62] Strong reactions to the Pfizer or Moderna vaccines, such as experiencing a flu for several days, are most likely with the second shot, when it fully activates immune response.[63] Strong reactions were experienced after just one shot by people previously infected with SARS2, a huge problem if estimates are correct that for each known infection, four times that number had already been infected. This was so concerning that some scientists suggested that these patients forgo the second shot.[64]

Given these results, and the problems of translating vaccine trials from small numbers to mass populations, and the observation period shortened by the FDA from three months to two, one wonders about how mass vaccinations can safely occur far away from emergency rooms. Scott Gottlieb proposed letting CVS and Walgreens drug store chains give shots, but what happens there when someone has a severe allergic reaction?[65] Will an EpiPen be enough? Do they need ambulances on standby? "We are really pushing to make sure that anybody administering vaccines needs not just to have the EpiPen available but, frankly, to know how to use it," said Dr. Nancy Messonnier, director of the CDC's National Center for Immunization and Respiratory Diseases.[66] Severe reactions may require oxygen, antihistamines, and steroids given with intravenous lines, which staff in remote areas may not have.

Recall that during the Spanish flu of 1918–20, how the media reported on that flu raised ethical issues, especially when newspapers downplayed the seriousness of the disease during World War I. Similarly, the early rollout of the Pfizer and Moderna vaccines saw some massaging of the truth by authorities, who appear to have downplayed severe reactions to these vaccines in order to encourage greater acceptance by the public. In another case, Anthony Fauci admitted to *New York Times* veteran reporter Donald McNeil that he had not told Americans what he really thought about herd immunity and did not do so "until the country was ready to hear what he really thinks."[67] Fauci said, "When polls said only about half of all Americans would take a vaccine, I was saying herd immunity would take 70 to 75 percent. Then, when newer surveys said 60 percent or more would take it, I thought, 'I can nudge this up a bit, so I went to 80, 85.'"[68]

A day or so later, the *New York Times* reported in detail for the first time that two volunteers in the clinical trials for the Pfizer and Moderna vaccines had experienced problems considerably more significant than had previously been reported. Indeed, previous reports make both the effects of taking either vaccine seem milder than taking seasonal flu shots, with many public pronouncements of "I felt nothing more than a little arm soreness," but in reality, 16 percent of those receiving the first shot of the Moderna vaccine "had a reaction strong enough to prevent them from going about their daily routine." After a first shot, one ER doctor said she spent the day after vaccination "in a mental fog that turned her attempt at the most basic of meals into an inedible blob," and another doctor was up all night with a fever, alternating with feeling extremely cold, while another had 36 hours of a bad headache and nausea.[69] After taking the vaccine, most physicians and nurses hesitated to share news of any bad after-effects for fear of discouraging others, especially from the second dose, which seemed to create more severe after-effects.[70] Reports on social media of adverse effects led about one third of North Americans to wait and see before getting vaccinated.

AstraZeneca experienced a setback in March 2021 when a dozen European nations paused its rollout after reports of fatal blood clots emerged in about 18 people. After an investigation, European officials concluded that this rate of fatal clots was not higher than usual, and the rollout of AstraZeneca's vaccine continued, albeit with some suspicion in some quarters. The next month, a UK advisory board said the vaccine should not be given to people under 30 because of the clots. During the same month, the United States paused Johnson & Johnson's vaccine after six women experienced the rare blood-clotting disorder cerebral venous sinus thrombosis (CVST), which creates clots in the blood vessels of the brain. One woman died and another was hospitalized in critical condition.[71] Neither of these vaccines used the mRNA technology of the Pfizer or Moderna vaccines but were instead viral vector vaccines.[72] Given that Johnson & Johnson's vaccine was one shot and AstraZeneca's was cheap and easy to store, these reactions set back worldwide vaccinations and increased skepticism about the safety of these vaccines.

This all raises the issue of media ethics, that is, whether physicians and leaders should tell the public the unvarnished, real truth about germs during pandemics or whether the public can stand to hear only so much truth and needs to be given it in small increments. The problem with the latter strategy is that as soon as smart people realize what's going on, they may cease trusting any of the pronouncements of public authorities.

MANDATORY VACCINATIONS

Mandatory Vaccination as Government Policy

If the greater good justifies human challenge trials, might it also justify mandatory vaccination of healthy adults? Three professors from law, medicine, and bioethics at Case Western Reserve University championed mandatory vaccination in the United States, arguing that national herd immunity could only be achieved this way.[73] They would deny religious objections to vaccination, stating that "the major religions do not oppose vaccinations," and would deny personal objections because such objections "violate the social contract." To get high vaccination rates, they think governments should refuse tax credits and some government benefits to vaccine refusers. Health insurers should charge them higher premiums. Schools should not admit unvaccinated children. What about citizens who travel or work in different places? These same professors propose a national "certification card" with an expiration date for everyone in the country, whether "here legally or not." As in China, without vaccination or an "immunity passport," North Americans couldn't fly, take a train, or ride a bus. Although the authors know their proposals might seem draconian, they conclude that the alternative, a sustained pandemic, is unacceptable.

Is this really possible? In a country where many people resist even wearing a mask? Invasion by the state of one's body is an ethical line that many hope will rarely be crossed, and being required by the state to inject an unknown substance into your body is a violation that could be justified only by a much greater, compensating good. What would constitute that greater, compensating good? First, the vaccine would need to be highly effective, such that one dose conferred a high degree of immunity for one or two years. Second, the vaccine would need to be very safe, having been tested on every ethnic group, gender, and age, and then found to have no harm. But what if, like the vaccine for Dengue fever, it made some people worse off? If that were true, mandatory vaccination would be hard to justify.

But don't we vaccinate all children?[74] The justification for doing so is utilitarian: vaccinating every child protects not only the child but other children in the community as well. Mandatory vaccination of children, say against measles, creates herd immunity, protecting vulnerable children with compromised immune systems who cannot get vaccines. Such a justification is rational and altruistic, but not every parent is rational and altruistic, so some parents refuse to vaccinate their children. Also, what is true for children is not necessarily true for adults. Mandatory vaccination of adults might create resistance in them, such as active rebellion against local ordinances and taking active measures to avoid vaccination. As a result, requiring vaccination might actually lead to lower rates of vaccination in populations such as France, where people are already deeply skeptical of vaccines. Covid hits African Americans especially hard, so they are prime candidates for a good vaccine, but many African Americans do not trust the federal government when it comes to medical research.[75] Wouldn't *forcing* them to take vaccines against their will be a bad idea?

What about colleges? Is it permissible for them to require vaccination against Covid for all students? Many already require vaccination for their students against mumps, rubella, and measles. In the spring of 2021, a dozen colleges already announced policies of mandatory vaccination for students returning to campus in the fall, including Duke, Cornell, Brown, Harvey Mudd, Johns Hopkins, and Notre Dame.

Nevertheless, two polls taken the previous summer found that one-third of college-age students would decline a vaccination for Covid.[76] Only 22 percent of Black college students and 37 percent of Hispanic students said they would take a Covid vaccine. Anti-vaxxer groups such as Children's Health Defense, founded by Robert Kennedy Jr., and Texans for Vaccine Choice, have vigorously opposed mandated COVID vaccines.[77] In late 2020, the Equal Employment Opportunity Commission ruled that employers must allow religious objections to vaccination, where "religious" includes "moral and ethical beliefs as to what is right and wrong," unless—and this is a crucial condition—allowing such exceptions would cause the business "undue hardship," which one Supreme Court defined as anything more than a minimal cost.[78]

Finally, until vaccines get approval for regular, non-emergency use, mandatory vaccinations will face significant legal challenges.[79] Because the safety data under Emergency Use Authorizations are less rigorous than that required for full Biologics License Application approval, those who are vaccine-hesitant or vaccine-resistant could argue that the FDA and government were overstepping Congressional authorization and that a specific new law allowing mandatory vaccinations should be passed at the federal or state level.

Mandatory Vaccination in Industry

As vaccines start to work and as pressures increase from economic shut-downs, policymakers start to ask about mandatory vaccination, which, as we saw in the previous section, raises many ethical issues. For example, should an employer require vaccination before employees enter a workplace? In 1905, the US Supreme Court decided that states could protect the public health by requiring the small-pox vaccination, even though that vaccination made some people sick.[80] Various vaccine experts, such as Paul Offit, think that vaccines need to be mandatory because "it's your responsibility as a citizen" to take it."[81]

So could employers in 2021 require employees to be vaccinated as a condition of working? In the United States, the answer is yes. Already medical centers and hospitals require employees to take standard vaccines, even seasonal flu vaccines, because otherwise they might spread germs to patients and to other employees. In 2021, two of the biggest American companies involved in operating long-term care homes required their employees, if they wanted to keep their jobs, to be vaccinated.[82] What about the 13 million manufacturing workers in the United States? Again, yes: employers could legally require vaccination, and ethically, in order to protect all workers, it could be justified for the same reason.

The analogy with measles vaccination and offices of pediatricians resonates here. Many pediatricians won't see children whose parents refuse to vaccinate their children against measles, which is highly infectious (such parents believe the vaccines are harmful). Pediatricians see children who are immune-compromised and who therefore can't take the vaccine and thus who are vulnerable to measles from unvaccinated children in their offices. To protect such vulnerable children, all children seeing the pediatrician must get vaccinated.

One legal exception to mandatory vaccination would be related to people with disabilities for whom the vaccination might make their disability worse. These people are covered under Title 7 of the Americans with Disabilities Act (ADA). Already some long-serving employees have sued their employers for forcing them to work on-site, rather than at home, when the employee contracted Covid and was seriously ill for months.[83] Note that fear of adverse effects is not enough to qualify for exemption under the ADA; real harm from vaccination must be proven.

What about airlines, most of which already required passengers to wear masks during the Covid pandemic? Certainly, where countries require proof of vaccination or negative PCR tests for SARS2, you can't get on an international flight if you can't get off. And if everyone else on the plane has been vaccinated, to protect crew and immune-compromised passengers, vaccination of the last person on that plane would be justified, eliminating free-riders (on which, see the next chapter). What about colleges? Again, many colleges now require various vaccinations before students enter campuses. A vaccine against a coronavirus is merely another step. Especially in this day of online and remote courses, students who won't take vaccinations can take courses in other ways. In the same way, employers need not fire employees who won't vaccinate but could offer them remote work or unpaid leave.

The metaphor of the carrot and stick helps here. Mandatory vaccination means forcing some people to have a needle stuck in their body against their will, by a stranger who injects a foreign substance into tissues and where they cannot be certain how they will react, an act that people in freedom-loving democracies only want to take as a last resort. Before that, incentives might work far better to achieve herd immunity. For example, suppose that only people who could prove they've been vaccinated would be admitted to concerts or theme parks such as Disney World. Such requirements would powerfully motivate vacillating people to get their shots. One can also predict that dating apps or employment agencies will make prospective partners prove they are vaccinated.

On the other hand, if Dr. Fauci is correct that herd immunity for SARS2 will require nearly 90 percent of people to be protected against the virus, either by vaccination or infection, then that figure may never be achieved without mandatory vaccination.

GLOBAL VACCINE DISTRIBUTION

Vaccine Nationalism versus Vaccine Globalism

In an extraordinary development under Operation Warp Speed, the Trump administration in 2020 paid $12 billion for vaccine production and ownership of six experimental vaccines.[84] For 100 million doses each, it paid $2 billion to Moderna,[85] $2 billion to Pfizer/BioNTech,[86] $2.1 billion to Sanofi and Glaxo-SmithKline, and $1.6 billion to a little-known company in Maryland, Novavax.[87] Amazingly, neither Moderna nor BioNTech had ever produced a vaccine, but both used the promising new RNA technology.

Canada followed, purchasing enough vaccines to vaccinate every Canadian six times, a move criticized by Amnesty International, which said Canada had secured many more doses than it needed, depriving other countries of them.[88] Britain and the European Union followed, buying enough vaccines to respectively inoculate everyone in their territories four times and two times over. Not wanting to be left out, Japan purchased rights to 120 million doses of Pfizer's vaccine.[89] The Serum Institute of India, a major manufacturer of vaccines, secured priority of vaccines made there for Indians. In this race to hoard vaccines, famous billionaire Carlos Slim secured millions of doses for his home countries of Argentina and Mexico.

Canada, the United States, and Japan purchased vaccines only for their citizens. Those in developing countries such as Bolivia and Uganda wondered when, if ever, they might get their vaccines. Already the wealth gap had been growing across the globe, and the unequal distribution of Covid vaccines threatened to worsen that gap. If the coronavirus stays around for years, it could take until the end of 2024 for poorer countries to get enough vaccine to cover citizens of their countries.[90] "The worst possible outcome is you're offering vaccines to a whole country's population before we're able to offer it to the highest risk ones in other countries," said Dr. Bruce Aylward, who works with WHO's global vaccine program.[91] In stark contrast to the practices of some of the world's large and powerful nations, the vaccine being developed by the non-profit Jenner Institute at Oxford University, in partnership with AstraZeneca, would be given out freely to essential workers in all countries, not just to citizens of Britain.[92]

The Jenner Institute practices *vaccine globalism* because it is working for all humans on the planet, not just citizens of Britain. In contrast, *vaccine nationalism* occurs when one country buys a vaccine exclusively for its own citizens. David Heymann, a fellow at London's Chatham House Global Health program, says, "Most countries are going to be politically obliged to make sure it [the successful vaccine] goes to their own people if it's being produced and manufactured in their own country."[93] The United States bought Pfizer's vaccine for $2 billion and gave Moderna $2 billion for first rights to its vaccine to try to guarantee that Americans were vaccinated first.[94]

Vaccine nationalism appeared when Britain actually beat the United States in administering Pfizer's vaccine, with the UK's secretary of education boasting that Britain had beaten the United States and Europe because "we've obviously got the best medical regulators," a statement that made British scientists cringe and led to a challenge by Anthony Fauci. Fauci countered that British regulators had not as carefully scrutinized the data for Pfizer's clinical trials as the FDA had, which, he emphasized, were the "gold standard" of such regulation.[95]

The leader of vaccine globalism for Covid is the GAVI Alliance, formerly known as the Global Alliance for Vaccines and Immunization.[96] GAVI already united the WHO, the World Bank, the Gates Foundation, and private donors to vaccinate half the children in developing countries. For Covid, it hopes to distribute 2 billion dosages of the AstraZeneca vaccine to medical and essential workers around the world. It endorses Covid Vaccines Global Access (Covax), an effort by the WHO and GAVI to fairly distribute any successful vaccine for Covid across the planet.[97] As of August 2020, 160 nations had signed up to cooperate with GAVI. The United States under the Trump administration declined to commit vaccines to GAVI, but the Biden administration reversed that decision and did in fact pledge some.[98] Meanwhile, AstraZeneca's CEO has repeatedly promised that it will not profit from its vaccine and has set a target to make 2 billion doses.[99]

By spring 2021, Covax had secured only about a half billion doses of various Covid vaccines for the 4 billion people in developing countries.[100] Moderna priced its two-dose vaccine at $64–74 and Pfizer/NBiotech at $39, while Astra-Zeneca has said it will charge its cost, that is, between $3 and $4.[101] Critics have wondered why the public should allow Big Pharma to profit from vaccines that the public had financed, but that is also true for many devices and drugs, funded for discovery by NIH, which then allows drug companies to patent, sell, and profit from these creations. Pfizer, for its part, did not accept government money for the development of its vaccine: the $1.9 billion it received from Operation Warp Speed was merely an advance purchase. Also, partly because of pressure from champions of developing nations, Moderna said that, as long as the pandemic lasts, it wouldn't fight developing nations for infringement of its patents on its Covid vaccine and the technology to make it.[102]

Even if they vaccinated every one of its citizens, which is doubtful and even if they achieved a transient, mild herd immunity, could the United States and Canada immunize themselves against the coronavirus without helping the rest of the globe do so too? Can one continent wall itself off from others? The modern world is a very interconnected place where millions of North American businesspeople and tourists typically fly over the globe each year, and millions of tourists visit North America from other countries.

Pope Francis has repeatedly opposed vaccine nationalism, both in his 2021 Easter address and before. In his 2020 Christmas address, he said,

> We cannot allow the various forms of nationalism closed in on themselves to prevent us from living as the truly human family that we are.... Nor can we allow the virus of radical individualism to get the better of us and make us indifferent to the suffering of other brothers and sisters.... I cannot place myself ahead of others, letting the law of the marketplace and patents take precedence over the law of love and the health of humanity.[103]

In a similar criticism, the WHO's director general warned of a "catastrophic moral failure" if rich countries hoarded vaccines for themselves.[104] While Canada and the United States ordered enough vaccines to vaccinate their citizens many times over, poor countries such as Guinea got "not 25 million, not 25,000, but just 25 dosages for their entire country."[105]

Because of the anti-vaxxer movement and because of concerns about vaccine safety, a third of Americans might refuse a vaccine created under Operation Warp Speed.[106] This means that the unvaccinated third would still be susceptible to infection from any visitors to the country, or if they traveled overseas. Ultimately, only a worldwide approach can stop the Covid pandemic, just as it took a worldwide approach to eliminate the smallpox virus from the globe in 1980.[107]

Big Pharma and Big Biotech versus the Developing World

In November 2020, developing nations led by South Africa and India asked the WHO to suspend the patent rights of Big Pharma on successful vaccines so they could make the vaccines at home.[108] Another block of developed nations, led by the United States and including Japan and the European Union, opposed them.

A much larger philosophical issue lies beneath the specific issue of access to a Covid vaccine, and that is how intellectual property should be protected across the globe. On one side are free-market globalists who think an expanding world economy benefits all countries and who believe that patents motivate inventors to create valuable, new products, for which they can charge and make profits. Because of such profits, investors buy stocks in companies funding research into new drugs, new kinds of seeds, and new vaccines. On the other side are those who believe that all intellectual property, such as music, books, art works, software, and scientific discoveries, should belong to the world and not be patented, copyrighted, or legally protected from infringement. In medicine, the debate involves not only money but also lives and health, for denying access to patented medicines can cause loss of life.

On November 24, 2020, the WHO celebrated the 25th anniversary of the Agreement on Trade-Related Aspects of Intellectual Property Rights (TRIPS), which protects intellectual property from being stolen—such as patents on drugs and devices, as well as copyright of books, songs, and art.[109] The US Founding Fathers cared so much about such protection of intellectual property that they put it in the US Constitution (Article 1, Section 8, Clause 8 gives Congress the power "to promote the Progress of Science and Useful arts, by securing, for limited Times, to Authors and Inventors, the exclusive Right to their respective Writings and Discoveries"). However, during the AIDS crisis, activists got Big Pharma to allow production of cheap, generic, anti-retroviral drugs against AIDS for the developing world in a process known as compulsory licensing.[110] Also, in 2001 the WHO affirmed the Doha Declaration on the Agreement on Trade-Related Aspects of Intellectual Property Rights and Public Health, which affirmed that patent rules could be interpreted and implemented to protect public health and to promote access to medicines for all. Since Doha, more than 60 developing countries have procured large quantities of generic versions of patented medicines.[111] South Africa has argued that the WHO should allow developing countries access to patents on vaccines and the right to make copies without paying exorbitant fees.

The United States holds the patent on a key process for developing mRNA vaccines that allows scientists to swap a pair of amino acids on the spike protein of a coronavirus.[112] The patent was developed by years of NIH-funded work by American scientist Barney Graham, and developing nations want the United States to grant everyone public access to that patent (and process), allowing them to make cheap mRNA vaccines. But the major pharmaceutical companies oppose such a move.

The cost of vaccines will not be an issue in rich countries, which are generally providing them free to their citizens, but it will be an issue in other countries. As noted above, Pfizer is charging the US $39 for its two doses. One solution is a tier structure, setting one price for rich countries, another for middle-income countries, and the lowest price for the poorest nations. Even with such pricing, it might take years to vaccinate people in poor countries. Because of vaccine nationalism and because developing countries may not receive enough vaccines to cover their populations until the end of 2024, lack of vaccines there would create huge reservoirs of SARS2, crippling economies and deepening global inequality. Even Canada, which had no capacity to produce vaccines, had to wait in line for its 20 million doses of Pfizer's vaccine, conceding that the countries that had manufactured the vaccines would cover their citizens first.

In this controversy, Bill Gates and his Gates Foundation have urged that rich countries such as Saudi Arabia and the United States join Covax, which most declined to do. Nevertheless, the Gates Foundation has $50 billion to use to purchase Covid vaccines, and it looks like it might do so.[113] Spokespeople for pharmaceutical companies have pushed back, arguing that such companies need patent protection to incentivize their scientists and investors to develop future vaccines. They note that during the Covid pandemic, AstraZeneca, Johnson & Johnson, and GlaxoSmithKline have all pledged to offer their vaccines at cost.[114] The former director of the WHO's Intellectual Property Organization even queried whether the attempts of India and South Africa to suspend patent protection of Covid vaccines weren't self-serving for their own manufacturers and designed to reveal trade secrets that would cripple the development of vaccines in the future.[115]

POSSIBLE BAD SCENARIOS

Bad Scenario #1: Politicized Allocation of Vaccines

Let us first look at how things can go wrong in distributing vaccines. A hint came when New York governor Andrew Cuomo said in 2020 that he would not take President Trump's word that a vaccine would be safe; instead, he wanted independent scientists to verify safety. When Pfizer's vaccine came out later, President Trump said he would not allocate vaccines to New York.[116] This threat was appalling, because it indicated that the president saw vaccines as patronage spoils that he could allocate to friends and deny to enemies, rather than as public goods needed by all Americans. In March, he had forced governors to curry favor with him to get ventilators and PPE in federal stockpiles. (Chapter 12 discusses issues of leadership during pandemics, and the leadership of President Trump specifically.) Although the president's threat was shocking, carrying it out would have been worse and would have *weaponized* the distribution of vaccines. This happened when the Ayatollah Ali Khamenei, Iran's supreme leader, banned the import in 2021 to Iran of American- and British-made vaccines in favor of Chinese and Russian vaccines.[117]

Why would it be foolish to distribute the vaccine only to states that voted for an incumbent party and deny it to states that voted for the other party? One reason is that viruses don't respect state lines, and neither do Americans. Truckers, pilots, traveling nurses, and vacationers visit different states, patronize restaurants and motels, and hence spread germs. Leaving some states without vaccinations would create reservoirs for the virus. This is also why vaccine nationalism won't stop a pandemic, because no nation can wall itself off forever.

Different versions of politicizing vaccines have occurred around the globe. Russia and China bragged about creating their own vaccines, faster than the West, but many scientists were skeptical. China's CoronaVac vaccine was tested in Brazil but was only 50-percent effective against Covid.[118] Almost every politician was guilty of creating unrealistic expectations about the time between the approval of a vaccine and getting it to citizens. Unfortunately, almost no country in the West created a national plan for the complex logistics of "the final mile" of distribution of vaccines.

Bad Scenario #2: Large Numbers Refuse Vaccination, Defeating Herd Immunity

Unfortunately, everything about the Covid pandemic in the United States became politicized, even taking vaccines. By the time Joe Biden was inaugurated in January 2021, many Trump supporters had refused to take the coronavirus seriously or wear masks, so they naturally believed that getting vaccinated wasn't necessary. After the Pfizer and Moderna vaccines came out, 42 percent of Republicans said they definitely would refuse the vaccines.[119] Two months later, one-quarter of Americans told pollsters they "definitely would not" or "probably would not" take any Covid vaccine.[120]

The name of the US program developing vaccines, Operation Warp Speed, also led many Americans to believe that the vaccines had been rushed and weren't safe. Indeed, despite Trump's taking credit for safe vaccines, Republicans often cited such concerns. Moreover, a dangerous trend had developed in American cultural and political wars: using social media to spread falsehoods. In California, a group of 50 protestors who had previously campaigned against masks and lockdowns pivoted to vaccine protests and disrupted a mass-vaccination site at Dodger Stadium.[121] So worrisome was this that Britain passed laws making it illegal to spread falsehoods about vaccines. In France, despite its being the home of the Pasteur Institute, 60 percent of its citizens distrusted Covid vaccines and said they would refuse one.[122]

On the other hand, given the news that began to trickle in about severe allergic reactions to the new vaccines approved for emergency use, was it irrational to wait and see what happened? It seemed premature to lump everyone with such reservations into the anti-vaxxer camp, as Chris Hayes of MSNBC appeared to do one night.[123] And there are religious issues. In Muslim countries such as Indonesia, some clerics doubted whether vaccines were Halal.[124] In the United States, various Catholic bishops urged followers to avoid vaccines that had been developed using cell lines originally derived from tissue of aborted fetuses, which seemed to be AstraZeneca and Johnson & Johnson vaccines, and indirectly, the Pfizer vaccine. In late February 2021, about half of the country's 41 million white evangelical Christians said they would refuse vaccination, citing beliefs that vaccines used aborted fetal tissue and contained dangerous, experimental biological agents; distrust of mainstream science; and religious fatalism ("It would be God's will if I am here or not here").[125]

The possibility of a large percentage of citizens refusing vaccination became a worse problem in late 2020 when Anthony Fauci, who in spring 2020 had previously estimated "60 to 70 percent" vaccination rate for herd immunity, delivered a stark message at the end of that year, after the science had changed, stating it might take a 90-percent US vaccination rate to halt the virus, as much as needed to stop an outbreak of measles.[126]

Bad Scenario #3: Vaccine Roll-Out Disasters

The job of "the last mile" of actually getting vaccines into arms was dumped on the states with no planning and no resources.[127] Because countries had never tried to vaccinate a whole country, especially with a two-dose vaccine, massive planning was necessary. In addition, citizens needed to be taught patience, and plans needed to be made about where and when vaccines could be obtained. Federal money had not reached states as of January 8, 2021, putting them in a difficult position. If vaccines were created at warp speed, communication about how they would be delivered was created at "no speed." Looking back, many states confidently predicted that they had developed rational plans for distributing vaccines,[128] but such plans assumed a perfect world, national planning, and fine coordination, as well as public agreement about priorities, none of which actually materialized.

Making the first vaccines turned out to be far easier than getting shots into arms. Instead of 20 million Americans getting two doses by the end of December as predicted, about 2 million got one dose. During the same time, Israel vaccinated 10 percent of its population, a half million of its 5 million. As the *New York Times* editorial board wrote, the US vaccine rollout was "an astonishing failure—one that stands out in a year of astonishing failures."[129] Alas, such failures have become agonizingly familiar to Americans: "Poor coordination at the federal level, combined with a lack of funding and support for state and local entities.... We have been here before...with testing. With shutdowns. With contact tracing. With genomic surveillance."[130]

Operation Warp Speed first allocated Pfizer and Moderna doses to states based on population.[131] Some states had a plan for the whole state; others gave the vaccine to counties or hospitals, which devised their own plans. Once thawed, the Pfizer vaccine had a very short life. When people failed to make appointments and lest the scarce vaccine be wasted, nurses had to scramble to find someone to vaccinate. Huge questions popped up immediately about, even if priorities could be established, how workers or patients with chronic problems would know it was their turn. Other questions emerged about liability for administering the vaccine (especially in Europe). In some cases, even workers in plants making vaccines were not considered essential workers and could not themselves get vaccinated.[132]

When the United States finally increased testing, after most other developed countries had done so, it ran into another problem: lack of reagents for the tests (which had been purchased by other countries). This scarcity delayed mass testing in the United States for many months. Similarly, when the Pfizer vaccine was created, it ran out of materials to make vaccines, so much so that when the United States wanted an extra 100 million doses, Pfizer required the country to promise to supply the ingredients. Europe, however, fared much worse. It had delayed signing contracts for vaccines and therefore had to wait behind other countries that had signed early. By late March 2021, when Israel, the United States, and Britain had a third of their citizens vaccinated, many European countries struggled to get 10 percent vaccinated, contributing to a "third wave" in Europe and necessitating more unpopular lockdowns. A loosely inspected factory in Baltimore, the main American factory that made the AstraZeneca and Johnson & Johnson vaccines, could not gain approval for its 150 million doses, and 15 million doses of the Johnson & Johnson vaccine had to be discarded in April 2021 because of contamination.

Bad Scenario #4: A Premature Return to Normal

After many people who've endured pandemic fatigue get vaccinated, they may revert to pre-pandemic behavior, thinking "Now I won't get sick or die." As one person said after his first shot, "Now I feel invulnerable!" They might assume they can no longer transmit germs to others. That may be false. They might be vaccinated against severe illness, but not against harboring virus. If substantial numbers of vaccinated people resume normal behavior—for example, attending concerts and sports events with tens of thousands close together—such behavior could lead to amplification systems for SARS2 and especially its variants. If variants with the Eek mutation prosper, North Americans and the world may be looking at annual booster shots targeting multiple variants or booster shots of their original vaccines.

Another possibility lies in the category of "Be careful what you wish for." If people work remotely from home, taking care of children or dressing as they wish, what happens when they are fully vaccinated? Can they be required to resume on-site work? What about teachers and professors who've been teaching from home on Zoom? Colleges want to resume on-campus classes as soon as possible because they make the most money from room and board. Will colleges require all fully vaccinated professors to immediately work on campus? What happens if professors get vaccinated, but their spouses and children need to wait six months? If good childcare is still lacking? Could professors bring the virus home and infect their families?

FINAL NOTE

No one in the Trump administration planned the rollout of any vaccine. New CDC Director Rochelle Wallensky immediately learned that the previous administration "had essentially lost track of 20 million vaccine doses that were delivered to the states."[133] Nor was it much solace that the European Union had not done better, being embroiled in disputes among its members that delayed initial contracts for vaccines and faced with both a risk-averse bureaucracy and massive vaccine hesitancy among its public—so much so that by April 11, 2021, a mere 2 percent of EU citizens had been vaccinated.[134] It was interesting that after the arrival of successful vaccines, critics on both the left and the right wondered why development couldn't have been faster, either through challenge studies or giving people experimental vaccines sooner.[135] Given how many people thought that Operation Warp Speed had whipped out vaccines too fast, these criticisms seemed misguided.

Suppose vaccines work, give recipients some immunity, and prevent transmission of the virus—all good things. Supposing this, we want the most people possible to be vaccinated, especially those who work face-to-face with customers. But how then do they prove they've been vaccinated? How do we tell if your co-workers have been vaccinated? Do we take their word? Should a national vaccination card be issued with a hologram to prove it? This is a topic in Chapter 10.

Finally, Moderna is doing more clinical trials to explore other ways to use its vaccine. At the start of 2021, it said it would take two months to decide whether lowering the recommended dosage or giving only one shot would produce the same results. Intriguingly, it is also exploring whether giving people a *third* shot of its vaccine can lengthen or strengthen immunity, either to Covid or to getting the virus.[136]

FURTHER READING

Offit, Paul. *Vaccinated: One Man's Quest to Defeat the World's Greatest Diseases.* New York: HarperCollins, 2005.

Plotkin, Stanley. *History of Vaccine Development.* Cham, Switzerland: Springer, 2011. [See also his paperback *On Vaccines* (independently published 2019, an inexpensive, self-published summary of his expensive *History*).]

Youngdahl, Karie, et al. *The History of Vaccines.* Philadelphia: College of Physicians, 2013.

CHAPTER 8
ACTS AND OMISSIONS, THE TROLLEY PROBLEM, AND PRISONER'S DILEMMAS

This chapter uses some classic tools from philosophy and bioethics that can illuminate ethical issues about Covid. It covers the acts and omissions doctrine, the Trolley Problem, the Prisoner's Dilemma, and briefly, the doctrine of double effect.

ACTS VERSUS OMISSIONS

The *acts and omissions doctrine* holds that omitting an action that leads to a bad result is less serious, or less wrong, than acting to create that bad result. Another way of putting this doctrine is that we are less responsible for our omissions than for our actions.[1] James Rachels rejected this doctrine in 1975, arguing that if a physician *intends* to let a patient die and the *result* is the patient's death, then actively killing the patient does not morally differ from omitting life-sustaining treatment.[2] For Rachels in both cases, the motive and results are death, and worse, letting die sometimes allows more suffering than killing.

One aspect of ethics captured by the acts and omission doctrine is that it *feels* different to kill someone than to let them die. Defenders of abstract reason retort that many of our feelings are irrational, and if we can do the most good by removing a ventilator from a dying patient and giving it to a more promising one, we should do so. Nevertheless, for the person deciding to remove the ventilator, it often feels like taking a life.

With terminal sedation, the *doctrine of double effect* enters the acts and omissions doctrine. According to it, and when applied to mercy-killing, an action having two effects, one good and the other evil, is morally permissible if physicians intend only the good effect, not the bad effect—for example, to relieve suffering, not to kill. Lawyers defending Dr. Anna Pou at Memorial Hospital in New Orleans after Hurricane Katrina used it to argue that she intended only the good effect of relieving suffering (by administering morphine and other drugs), rather than the death of her patients. Critics point to Dr. Jack Kevorkian's use of the same defense, where after 100 similar mercy killings, judges had no doubt that Kevorkian intended more than relief of suffering. Kant would object that once you open the door to physicians' killing their patients, for initially compassionate reasons, we open a Pandora's Box where less virtuous physicians will kill undesirable patients.

In the Covid world, it may be impossible to treat every Covid patient with the highest standards of care: there aren't enough ICUs, PPE, ventilators, alert physicians, or nurses to do so. After a year of Herculean efforts, staff at hospitals with many Covid patients were often exhausted and burned out, and many quit. In this situation, when does not giving the highest standard of care amount to not giving the normal standard of care? And when does not giving the normal standard of care amount to tacitly letting a Covid patient die? And is a tacit decision to let a Covid patient die the same as killing that patient? Defenders of the distinction would answer negatively, arguing that Covid is killing the patient, not the exhausted staff. Also, humans have finite amounts of care that they can give when faced with mass infections during pandemics. But if tacit decisions are made to let a Covid patient die, is Rachels correct that, in some cases, killing them would be more humane than letting the agonizing process of suffocation kill them? Because SARS2 attacks the lungs, many terminal Covid patients felt like an elephant was sitting on their chests, making them struggle for each breath. If 99 percent of 95-year-old Covid patients in the ICU never leave the hospital, and if the staff have a 95-year-old patient who is slowly deteriorating, is it wrong to make that patient's final time one of days rather than weeks? If the patient arrests, can CPR be forgone, even if they have not signed a DNR order?

Overall, discussion of the acts and omission doctrine in Covid world, which unfortunately we have only begun here, maps a range of responsibility, guilt, compassion, and possible actions, from ideal and supererogatory to standards of care in normal, non-pandemic times, to evolving standards during a pandemic with massive increases in patients, and then to judgments at the end of life about medical futility and humane dying.

THE TROLLEY PROBLEM

In recent years, the *Trolley Problem* has been used to illustrate dilemmas regarding moral responsibility and decision making. Consider a runaway trolley in San Francisco speeding down the tracks of a steep hill. The trolley races straight for five people below, who have been tied up and cannot move. You are a bystander standing beside the track, next to a lever. If you pull this lever, the trolley will switch to a different set of tracks containing only one person. You have two options: (1) Do nothing and allow the trolley to kill five people; or (2) Pull the lever, divert the trolley, and kill one person. This version of the Trolley Problem is called "Bystander at the Switch."

The dilemma originates in Philippa Foot's classic article, "The Problem of Abortion and the Doctrine of Double Effect."[3] As one book about Foot and the Trolley problem explains,

> ... Philippa Foot described a group of spelunkers deciding whether to dynamite a companion stuck in the only exit from a flooding cave, a judge hanging an apparently blameless suspect to save more innocents from a bloody-minded mob, a pilot whose airplane is going down choosing to aim for a more or less populated area, a doctor who could kill a healthy individual to produce a serum or obtain body parts to save several patients from death, and, fatefully, the driver of a runaway tram whose vehicle will strike and kill five workmen unless he steers it onto another track where it will kill only one workman.[4]

Foot asked this question: What is the significant moral difference between the bystander directing the trolley away from five people even if it will thereby plow into another person, and surgeons not extracting organs from one healthy person to save five lives?

Today, the Trolley Problem uses hypothetical scenarios where runaway trams or "trolleys" may be diverted to save more people by sacrificing fewer, exploring whether causing such sacrifices to occur is worse than merely observing them and doing nothing. The Trolley Problem has even been featured on the cable television show *The Good Place*.[5] Since Foot's essay (and Judith Jarvis Thomson's and Frances Kamm's subsequent expansions of this thought experiment[6]), the Trolley Problem has fascinated moral philosophers and, more recently, psychologists and neuroscientists. The Trolley Problem reveals how we have inherited conflicting moral intuitions from different historical ethical theories and how even our non-theoretical moral intuitions may conflict. Foot herself thought that the bystander should not hesitate to redirect the tram, whereas the doctor and the judge should not take the life of an innocent person.

During the Covid pandemic, moral choices akin to those of the Trolley Problem appeared when all the ICU beds were full and when all ventilators were in use. Remember Nurse Jones, who knows that two patients in their 20s, George and Brianna, wait in the emergency room for admission while one of her elderly patients, Sam, will probably not last the week. Sam, at age 85, has underlying diabetes and cardiac arrythmias, and is overweight. From the perspective of triage and utilitarianism, Nurse Jones should remove Sam's ventilator, give him extra morphine, and let him struggle to live without further medical aid. But removing Sam's ventilator, or even simply taking him from the sophisticated equipment and intensive staffing of the ICU to a standard room, *feels* to Nurse Jones like she's taking his life. Is this irrational?

In the Bystander version of the Trolley Problem, someone is going to die whatever the bystander does. The bystander hasn't caused the trolley to lose its brakes or the people below to be placed where they are. If the bystander does nothing, five people die. If she acts, only one dies. Surely, she can't be blamed for saving four lives? Even if she pulls the switch to save the lives of five, she may feel some remorse over the death of the innocent person who is subsequently killed. After all, but for her actions, that person would be alive and given the fact that there was a runaway trolley, none of the five could claim as their right that the Bystander must save them. If she just froze in indecision, and the trolley killed the five, few would consider the bystander a bad person.

Now consider the Large Tourist variation of the Trolley Problem. A large tourist wearing a heavy backpack has stopped on a bridge that crosses parallel to the tracks below. A runaway trolley below has one track with five people bunched together ahead. In this case, the bystander could push the large man onto the tracks below, and his weight with the backpack would stop the train and save the five people. Most people think it's wrong to push the large man over the bridge, but why?

One thing that seems to matter morally is being the direct agent of another person's death by actively pushing that person to his death. Foot argued that it was permissible to re-direct an existing threat that necessarily will kill those on one track or the other, but it is entirely different to sacrifice an innocent person who otherwise is not involved and who otherwise would not be killed. In a similar medical case, she imagined a drug that might either save one patient with a very large dose or save five patients with a small dose. In this example, she thought the physicians should save the five patients. On the other hand, she thought it wrong to excise the organs from an innocent person to save five others waiting for an organ transplant.[7]

The Trolley Problem, Variolation, and the Dengvaxia Vaccine

The Trolley Problem illustrates the ethical problems of vaccination, because those giving the vaccines know that a small number of people getting vaccinated will get sick or even die from bad reactions to the vaccine, but overall, the vaccines will save many more people. Recall the example from Chapter 6 of the dengue virus (DENV) and Dengue fever.[8] According to the WHO, in the southern parts of Asia and much of Latin America, Dengue fever still kills 9,000 children and severely sickens 3.2 million each year.[9] The WHO recommends that only children older than nine be given the Dengvaxia vaccine, on the assumption that almost all of them had been previously exposed to some variant of DENV and hence would not be in the minority of DENV-virgins.

To review what went wrong, recall from Chapter 6 that because some Filipino children hadn't been exposed to one of the virus's four variants, Dengvaxia actually made some worse off. According to a report in the *New England Journal of Medicine*, "the vaccine is protective among those previously exposed but increases the risks of hospitalizations and severe illness among the unexposed."[10] What may have occurred is that Dengvaxia made the immune systems of those never exposed to DENV hyper-respond to exposure to DENV, probably because the vaccine produced cytokine storms. As noted, some such hyper-responsive children became so sick that they needed hospitalization, and some, unfortunately, died. Nevertheless, for over 800,000 children, Dengvaxia reduces severe sickness and death by 80 percent, so using a utilitarian calculus, all these children should get the vaccine.

If you are the utilitarian bystander at the switch of this Trolley Problem, you administer Dengvaxia to all children over age nine, accepting the loss of some unexposed children, even though the vaccine may cause their deaths. If you don't, you're like the bystander who does nothing and watches the Trolley slam into five people, killing them, when you could have diverted it to kill only one. Are your hands cleaner because you did nothing? Is not vaccinating 400 million people each year and letting 3.2 million children get sick ethically permissible? Allowing 9,000 to die when, if all were vaccinated, only a few hundred might die?

Here someone might ask: Why not vaccinate only those children already exposed to DENV? Two problems exist here: many infections with DENV are asymptomatic, and no point-of-care test exists to measure prior exposure to DENV. All such tests must be sent to a laboratory and then doctors must wait for the results. In practice in the real world, no way exists to vaccinate only the children who have already been exposed to DENV.

The Trolley Problem and Covid Lockdowns

Lockdowns instantiate the Trolley Problem. Innocent patients, whom the virus will kill if society has no lockdowns, correspond to the innocent person on one track; the other track holds all the harm done by lockdowns, which may be more harmful than a pandemic's germ, and corresponds to the five innocent people. In this analogy, the bystander authorities divert the trolley away from the innocent patients via lockdowns, inflicting harm on the masses. It's intuitive that keeping people isolated prevents infection spread, but as explained in Chapter 4, lockdowns could actually cause *more* harm in sub-Saharan African countries, for example. Analogous to the Trolley Problem, the harms of the lockdowns are willed, whereas those of the virus are unwilled. Notice that no matter which track they choose, authorities must accept some foreseeable harms.

The Trolley Problem applies to a young country such as Niger, which may adopt either the Swedish approach or limited Focused Protection, deliberately allowing infection of its fragile seniors to spare harms to its masses of young. Especially in Central Africa, which as of spring 2021 has not yet been hit hard, the coming coronavirus is like a runaway trolley, and bystander authorities must quickly decide whether it will hit seniors or the young. Will they push many young, large tourists with backpacks off the bridge? Or let the trolley hit their seniors on the tracks below?

Does this analogy hold? In the original trolley variant, the large tourist pushed over the bridge must die to save the five, but in Niger, the outcomes are less certain because most of the young will not die and some seniors will die naturally, regardless of Covid. On the other hand, if lockdowns crash the economy, famine and murder will skyrocket, along with the other harms of lockdowns, so vast numbers of the young will be hurt badly. In analogical reasoning, the strength of the conclusion depends on the fit between the two things compared. Perhaps the comparison is too loose here between runaway trolleys and runaway viruses.

The Trolley Problem also has a version in media ethics. As with the vaccine for Dengue Fever, we know that some people who receive Covid vaccinations will have allergic reactions; some may even experience anaphylactic shock. When in April 1947 New York City vaccinated 2 million people against smallpox, authorities waged a huge public campaign to scare New Yorkers into lining up for the vaccine. When some people had adverse reactions, the media did not report them or implied that these people were hypochondriacs.[11] Was that justified? Is it permissible not to warn everyone of possible severe reactions in order to get the greatest possible number of people vaccinated? By doing so, aren't editors indirectly sacrificing a small number of people to the greater good? Of course, the more this happens, the more people distrust the media. It may be true, then, as Sir Walter Scott wrote in his poem *Marmion* in 1808, "Oh what a tangled web we weave, / When first we practise to deceive."

PRISONER'S DILEMMAS AND VACCINATION UPTAKE

For better or worse, most people getting vaccines are self-interested. Modern citizens understand the benefits of herd immunity, where 70 to 90 percent of the herd must be vaccinated and immune in order to protect everyone.[12] A classic problem enters the picture here: the *Prisoner's Dilemma*, a paradox about self-interest and cooperation.[13] Here is a version of the dilemma, known as "Honor among Thieves," from the *Stanford Encyclopedia of Philosophy*:

> Tanya and Cinque have been arrested for robbing the Hibernia Savings Bank and placed in separate isolation cells. Both care much more about their personal freedom than about the welfare of their accomplice. A clever prosecutor makes the following offer to each: "You may choose to confess or remain silent. If you confess and your accomplice remains silent, I will drop all charges against you and use your testimony to ensure that your accomplice does serious time. Likewise, if your accomplice confesses while you remain silent, they will go free while you do the time. If you both confess, I get two convictions, but I'll see to it that you both get early parole. If you both remain silent, I'll have to settle for token sentences on firearms possession charges. If you wish to confess, you must leave a note with the jailer before my return tomorrow morning."
>
> The dilemma faced by the prisoners here is that whatever the other does, each *individually* benefits more from confessing than they *both* benefit in jointly confessing. A common view is that the puzzle illustrates a conflict between group and individual *decision making*.[14]

In this case and in other examples of the Prisoner's Dilemma, each person has choices, but often the outcomes depend on what the others do. Similarly, in pandemics, each citizen has choices, but outcomes also depend on what others do.[15] Like Tanya and Cinque, each citizen has the option of cooperation or non-cooperation, or, put in stronger terms, doing their duty or betraying their fellow citizens. Everyone gains if each citizen wears a mask, physically distances in public, and frequently washes their hands. If most people follow these recommendations and free-riders do not, the free-riders also gain.

The concept of a *free-rider* enters the discussion here because some individuals may benefit from the action of others while doing nothing. Free-riders exist with vaccines because of herd immunity. Those who never get vaccinated benefit from herd immunity and are free-riders. The children of parents who never vaccinate against measles, which requires about 90 percent of children to be vaccinated for herd immunity, free-ride on the vaccinations of all other children. If 150 million Americans get infected and another 150 million get vaccinated, then the remaining 30 million Americans are relatively safe from infection and can be free-riders. (Of course, they would be taking a chance and could still get infected.)

The concept of free-riders also pertains to volunteers who test vaccines. After other vaccines become available, should a volunteer stay in their original trial?

Should they endeavor to discover if they received a placebo? If they originally enrolled hoping to get the experimental vaccine, are they obligated to stay in the trial long-term? If they do, aren't they the opposite of a free-rider?

Consider another example of unacceptable behavior by a free-rider, one that arises in a politically and culturally divided country, one where significant parts of the population accepted falsehoods that the coronavirus was not real, did not cause symptoms worse than the flu, and whose victims' deaths were faked or exaggerated. Now in any country, it is to everyone's advantage to know who is infectious and who might infect others, but notice what happens when a single Covid-denier takes a home-test for SARS2 and tests positive. Realizing now that her false beliefs have been exposed and that she may be perceived as a fool, what does she do? As a free-rider, she may tell no one and hope she will experience only mild symptoms. Of course, in doing so, she will need to act normally, interact normally with others, and probably infect others, who in turn will be mystified as to how they became infected. If she perceives it to be in her self-interest to remain free from ridicule and "I told-you-so" comments, she may keep her infection secret. As in the early weeks of the pandemic in New York and Italy, only if she becomes so sick that she needs to go to the emergency room will authorities know about her infection.

Researchers in game theory have used Prisoner's Dilemmas to model the uptake of vaccines, where self-interested citizens may hope to be free-riders on subsequent herd immunity. One thing they discovered is that acceptance of vaccines based purely on self-interest is lower than acceptance based on concern for others.[16] Second, and like classical economic theory, game theory assumes that rational self-interest governs behavior, but modern economists and game theory analysts have concluded that people do not always, or even usually, act purely from rational self-interest, so new fields have emerged, such as behavioral economics, that study how non-rational things motivate purchases and behavior.

Third, game theory also models two ways in which vaccines work: *direct and indirect protection*. Direct protection benefits the person vaccinated, whereas indirect protection benefits those around them. Most mass vaccination programs focus on direct protection, but in poor countries such as Niger or those with vast reservoirs of infection, game theory suggests that focusing on indirect protection would save more lives.[17] Moreover, as more glitches appear in the production of vaccines, or as resistance to taking vaccines grows, even Canada and the United States should continue to emphasize both indirect and direct protection, that is, do it for yourself and for those you care about.

Game-theory researchers have collaborated with psychologists to study what happens with uptake of vaccines when irrational factors enter. With vaccinations and using game theory, epidemiologists learned that even when overwhelming evidence exists that a vaccine is safe, fear can suppress acceptance of vaccinations, a phenomenon called *hysteresis* in physics and game theory. However, they also learned that creating feelings during a pandemic that "we're all in this together" could substantially increase the acceptance of vaccines.[18]

FURTHER READING

Edmonds, David. *Would You Kill the Fat Man? The Trolley Problem and What Your Answer Tells Us about Right and Wrong*. Princeton, NJ: Princeton University Press, 2014.

Kamm, Francis. *The Trolley Problem Mysteries*. Ed. Eric Rakowski. New York: Oxford University Press, 2015.

Poundstone, William. *The Prisoner's Dilemma: John von Neumann, Game Theory, and the Puzzle of the Bomb*. New York: Anchor, 1993.

CHAPTER 9
LIBERTY AND PRIVACY

Can Western democracies control pandemics? Can they grant generous liberties to their citizens and also fight infectious germs? Can they control contrarian behaviors and also protect privacy? This chapter explores these philosophical questions.

In recent history, Western democracies extolled individual rights, especially negative rights of non-interference. As Alasdair MacIntyre writes, in this sense individual political rights historically arose as limiting conditions against what the state could do to you.[1] In Canada and the United States, vast, open spaces allowed idiosyncratic individuals to roam and live as they wanted. Such a culture provides many advantages, especially for those who chafe against the normal manners of social life, such as not taking too much time to make a purchase when many others stand in line behind you. On the other hand, such a culture also makes it very difficult for officials to get citizens to act for the collective good.

Does this Western culture of rights overly promote individual freedom? In doing so, does it sacrifice the rights of the group? The family? The community? The nation? Does it impair our ability to respond to shared risks? Is it true that, in the East, they plan for 20 years down the road; in the West, we plan for Saturday night? Does Western culture celebrate individual achievement, while Eastern culture celebrates family, group, community, and national pride? Of course, that's an exaggeration, but it still stings.

The great personal liberty of citizens in the West presents a problem during pandemics, but in the long run, such liberty may triumph over other values. The control that China exercises over Hong Kong, or that Vladimir Putin exercises over Alexey Navalny and his followers, shows us how precious liberty is and how easily it can be lost. In many ways, tensions exist during pandemics between protecting individual liberty and protecting the most fragile.

PHILOSOPHICAL POSITIONS ON LIBERTY

Foucault on Domination and Control

Some famous philosophers claim that the state uses epidemics to seize new powers. For them, expertise in public health disguises a desire for *control*. The French philosopher Michel Foucault, for example, argued that elementary schools and hospitals exist to control those inside. The plight of captive populations during pandemics, such as those on aircraft carriers or in group homes, shows the extreme forms of state control over vulnerable groups. For Foucault, the state's every institution, from the military to police, from colleges to social workers, evolved to control people.[2]

Foucault emphasized that the hallmark of such control is to correct deviance, especially in individuals who are contrarian, who do not bend to the state's control. Rogues such as Jack Nicholson's character in the 1975 film version of Ken Kesey's *One Flew Over the Cuckoo's Nest* (1962) threaten the stability of mental institutions, so patients such as these must be drugged or lobotomized. In Aldous Huxley's 1932 novel *Brave New World*, the state distributes *soma* to tame citizens. Modern capitalism may have created more devious ways to exert similar controls: one in seven Americans aged 20 to 35 binge drinks once a week, while 80,000 Americans and thousands of Canadians die every year of opioid overdoses.[3] Meanwhile, Big Pharma convinces people that they cannot urinate, sleep, lose weight, defecate, or have sex without drugs. Television, sports events, movies, and highly structured religions induce mass numbness to control the populace.

For Foucault, not only do modern institutions exist to control people, but knowledge itself functions to do the same, especially in the way it categorizes people. In his *History of Madness*, Foucault describes how labels have functioned throughout history to control women, labels such as "witch," "bitch," "whore," "crazy," and "lesbian." For Foucault, madness is socially constructed to control deviance. This work fueled libertarian critiques of psychiatry, especially the 1962 book *Myth of Mental Illness*, by the Hungarian-American psychiatrist Thomas Szasz.[4]

Normally a philosopher's sexual orientation is irrelevant to his ideas, but not in Foucault's case. Like other gay men growing up in the early part of the twentieth century, Foucault learned to hide his homosexuality and believed that, because of it, the world was against him. In his four-volume *History of Sexuality*, written between 1976 and his death in 1984, Foucault considers pornography— which has always existed—as both a form of social control and categorization and a rebellion *against* social control.[5] Overall, practices and norms of the modern world strive to create pliant, docile bodies that must be trained, observed, and, above all else, rendered subservient to existing power.

More universally for Foucault, all institutions control people and their bodies in four basic ways: *spatially*, in how far apart bodies exist and intermingle; *organically*, forcing bodies into normal activities and suppressing abnormal actions; *genetically*, controlling the evolution over time of bodies and their offspring; and *combinatorily*, dictating when bodies can legitimately come together, such as groupings of police or military, students enrolled in a university, or agents of a national security agency. In *Discipline and Punish: The Birth of the Prison* (1975), Foucault traces the history of penal systems, which he believed to exist to turn inmates into objects that are predictable, docile, and pliant.

In summary, norms we see as natural for Foucault are socially constructed mechanisms for controlling deviance, normalizing individuals, and shaping how sexuality can be channeled into acceptable forms. What about science and medicine? For Foucault, it is difficult for societies to keep these things neutral. Modern physics is wonderful, but scientists used it to create atomic bombs. In medicine, the power of knowledge for Foucault is easily corrupted, as seen in medicine's centuries-long characterization of homosexuality, lesbianism, and intersex as psychiatric diseases that needed cures.

Foucault lived as he thought. He fought the controls on gay sexuality brought about to control HIV/AIDS and ultimately died of AIDS himself. So, during the Covid pandemic, his followers are willing to take the small risk of death by Covid to live freely. We might think of the behavior of 490,000 motorcycle riders who gathered at Sturgis, South Dakota, in the summer of 2020 as a striking example of this stance. Wearing masks, social distancing, avoiding large rallies, closing businesses, closing elementary schools and universities—Foucault would oppose all such measures, even focused protection, because he opposed any expansion of government control over citizens. For Foucault, once the state expands its powers during a pandemic, it rarely gives them back.

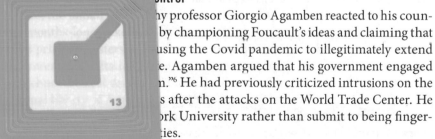

ontrol

y professor Giorgio Agamben reacted to his counby championing Foucault's ideas and claiming that using the Covid pandemic to illegitimately extend e. Agamben argued that his government engaged n."[6] He had previously criticized intrusions on the s after the attacks on the World Trade Center. He rk University rather than submit to being fingeries.

Foucault's and Agamben's views resonated in the fall of 2020 in Germany, where protests in Berlin drew 38,000 people protesting restrictions imposed by Chancellor Angela Merkel. In 2021, thousands of Dutch citizens protested in Amsterdam—unmasked and in large crowds without social distancing—against the strict controls imposed by the Netherlands.[7] Many of these protestors thought the virus no worse than a bad seasonal flu. Echoing Foucault and Agamben, these protests' leaders claimed that restrictions were designed to scare citizens and foster obedience to increased control; others called the pandemic a "Trojan Horse," designed to gain more power and liberties from citizens in the guise of disease protection.[8]

Especially for Agamben, getting infected with SARS2 is not worse than losing basic liberties. He also believes that most people under age 30 will either be asymptomatic or suffer very mild symptoms, and that only a small number of overweight, elderly men with other medical problems will die from Covid, at most 1–2 percent of the population. For Agamben, it's ridiculous to shutter economies to prevent such a small number of deaths, and more dangerously, it's wrong for the state to curtail individual liberties to do so. For those who agreed with him, not wearing facemasks symbolized resistance to unjust, government control.

Common to both Foucault and Agamben is their belief that knowledge confers power and how that power easily corrupts its bearer. Here they would move from content to process: Who decided to inflict great harm on billions of people to prevent a small number of Covid deaths? Who decided that kind of harm was a worthwhile tradeoff? Is corrupt political judgment hiding behind medical expertise? The tradeoff certainly entails both bioethical and political judgments. What kind of expertise is useful in making such judgments? As science writer Matt Ridley observes, "Where science becomes political, as in climate change and Covid-19, this diversity of opinion is sometimes extinguished in the pursuit of consensus to present to a politician or press conference and to deny the oxygen of publicity to cranks. This year [2020] has driven home as never before that there is no such thing as 'the science'; there are different scientific views on how to suppress the [SARS2] virus."[9]

Foucault and Agamben both ask us to take a wider view of controls started during pandemics and their wider repercussions. For example, do pandemic controls conceal class warfare? Do professionals who work at home to protect themselves from infection sacrifice the essential workers who service them? What about school children? The psychological trauma inflicted on tens of millions of children by paranoia about the virus and their stay-at-home schooling may damage them more than any virus. Who made these decisions and with what transparency? When will controls end and how?

Let us end this discussion of Foucault and Agamben with two comments. First, an obvious point: If a lethal germ is spreading in a country, *of course you want to control it*. If the behavior of your people increases the spread of that lethal germ, *of course you must modify that behavior* to better control the spread. Second, many have faulted Donald Trump for mishandling the Covid pandemic. Many worried that his narcissistic, chaotic style of governing came close to leading the United States into fascism. However, reading Foucault and Agamben makes us realize that had Trump used the pandemic as a guise to expand his power, he might have succeeded. Amazingly and fortunately, Trump did the opposite, minimizing the power of the federal government over the pandemic, downplaying the seriousness of the virus, and failing to intrude into the lives of citizens as much as his fellow leaders in Italy, New Zealand, and South Korea all did.

Libertarianism

Ideas similar to those of Foucault and Agamben frequently appeared in Libertarian thinking, a movement championed in analytic philosophy by Harvard philosopher Robert Nozick.[10] In American politics, the Libertarian Party sometimes elected candidates to public office, such as former Congressman Ron Paul (Texas), who mounted a real campaign for president in 2008 and 2012, and his son Rand Paul, an elected US Senator from Kentucky. Libertarians abhorred the harsh measures dictated by New York's governor Andrew Cuomo, citing his over-reach into personal liberties, his lack of accountability, and his distrust of building a consensus before acting. When several prominent restaurateurs left Manhattan for southern Florida to re-open, following thousands of rich citizens who had left that city for Florida, Libertarians felt vindicated.

Libertarianism has a long history in political philosophy, with branches on both the political left and the political right. However, all branches emphasize the primacy of individual liberties such as free movement and travel, free expression of ideas, free association, and protection of such rights from government control. As such, Libertarianism endorses almost all the ideas of Foucault and Agamben.

PROBLEMS OF CONTACT TRACING

In the context of this discussion of individual rights and control, we will now explore why contact tracing failed in the United States and why it worked in other countries, even in other democracies. Many assumptions underlie standard models of contact tracing used to slow the spread of infectious viruses—assumptions such as that professionals can spot the virus early, quickly develop tests for it, use those tests on at-risk people, discover who is positive, contact them about people they may have exposed, and contact those people so everyone will isolate and not infect others. Many of these assumptions are dubious, especially in North America and in other democratic countries that protect liberties.

As a public health strategy, tracing initiatives can feel intrusive to Westerners. These efforts rely on the tracer's attempt to locate the exposed individual and to document an individual's date of birth, address, and names of close contacts, including friends, family members, and sexual partners.[11] Preferably, contact tracing should be neither formulaic nor impersonal. Ideally, contact tracers build trust over several calls and build relationships by offering services and help, such as how to get paid during self-isolation or locating hotels where the exposed can stay at government expense. They might also help them find food or medicine. Later, the same contact tracers would hope to call infected people back and monitor their quarantine (and praise them for their adherence).

Ideally, contact tracers are evaluated not on how many calls they make a day or how many people answer but on how many contacts trust them. Instead, it appears that New York City's Test and Trace Corps was geared toward favorable publicity and metrics about how many people had been contacted.[12] When professional baseball teams in North America tried to resume play in the summer of 2020, two staffers on each team became in-house contact tracers.[13] In this context, the job is partly disease detective, partly therapist and friend, and partly social worker directing contacts to useful resources. The baseball league wanted to know which players were infected and whether they were cooperating, and the players wanted to be treated well, with respect, and not to be punished for getting sick.

One reason contact tracing works in countries with generous benefits is because workers there do not lose wages by self-isolating. Countries with successful contract tracers provided generous benefits for wages, housing, food, and medical supplies for those exposed and identified. New York City provided those exposed with free hotel stays and three meals a day for their 14-day monitoring period. Without such benefits for the exposed, contact tracers would have been in the untenable position of asking people to quarantine at their own expense—too much to ask for the public good, especially given that 40 million Americans were unemployed and many others worried about becoming so. New York City also gave those exposed the option of isolating at home and having essentials such as medical supplies and food delivered by the city. These services attempted to provide a level of respect toward the liberty, privacy, and autonomy of clients identified. All such quarantines and isolations, however, were voluntary, which meant that ultimately the programs failed.

In contrast, consider the case of Ashlyn Reynolds, employed at a restaurant near Richmond, Virginia, who felt slightly sick in July, got tested for SARS2, and had to wait 17 days *without pay* before getting a negative result.[14] With such delays, what's the point of contact tracing? Who can contract tracers ethically ask to voluntarily isolate without pay under such conditions?

Contact tracing assumed that when a stranger called, exposed people would answer their phones. Even lonely senior citizens, subjected to many junk calls and sales pitches, may not answer such calls. Even when they answer, Westerners may not cooperate: early contact tracers discovered that 58 percent of those infected New Yorkers whom they called between June 1 and July 25 never provided even a single contact.[15] Indeed, in New York City, with people coming from many different countries and speaking many languages, contact tracing for Covid went badly right away.[16] The city hired 3,000 people for its brand-new

Test and Trace Corps. Contact tracers were hired who could speak both English and French, but then were asked to call Spanish-speaking citizens.

There were no protocols for contacting infected people in nursing homes or hospitals, where staff were already overworked and taught to protect the privacy of patients. Additionally, protocols for new workers tracing infected children were confusing with respect to what to do with infected kids. Worse, during the first months of their job, the new contact tracers had to work through with those exposed a 45-minute questionnaire that included questions about sexual orientation, race, and ethnicity before they got to a question about whom they may have exposed to the virus. By this time, many of those called were fed up and refused to cooperate. Some who refused to cooperate were nonetheless called again several times by different contact tracers. And the contact tracers, largely working alone from remote locations, felt overwhelmed and untrained and had little confidence that they were doing any good.

On June 17, 2020, a crowd of 100 attended a party in a town north of New York City, and one of the partiers later tested positive for SARS2. However, it took court subpoenas to make eight of the attendees work with contact tracers.[17] In August, a bunch of parties attended by young people caused a flare-up of cases in Greenwich, Connecticut, but the partiers' parents refused to cooperate with contract tracers.[18] In such a system, and with such realities, contact tracing is difficult. Developing apps for contact tracing is also hard. For example, at the University of Alabama at Birmingham (UAB), an app developed by Apple and Google notified a student who had been near a Covid-positive person for more than 15 minutes, but it did not tell the student the names of such contacts (which the app knew).[19] The student would then supposedly self-quarantine for 14 days, either in his dorm room or at home. But the effectiveness of this system depended on an infected person truthfully revealing his infected status on his smart phone to UAB. It also depended on a student notified of exposure to have a phone in the first place, having that phone in good working order, switching on its GPS setting, and carrying the phone each day. Assume Jane is 20 years old and attending campus part-time while working as a waitress. Because of Covid lockdowns, she hasn't made enough money to pay her tuition and rent. Suppose she becomes infected, but like most people her age, she is asymptomatic. Suppose she wants to keep working because she fears not having money for rent, being evicted, and becoming homeless. Is Jane going to tell UAB or her restaurant about her infection? Wouldn't it be tempting for her to be a free-rider—to simply keep quiet and hope for the best?

More globally, contact tracing will work with some germs, but not others. With SARS2 creating asymptomatic but transmissible infections, and with some people having a "negative serial interval," meaning they showed signs before the person who had given it to them, contact tracing and isolation will not be enough to stop the spread of germs like SARS2.[20]

CONTROLLING PANDEMICS VERSUS PROTECTING PRIVACY

Philosophically, we might construct a graph with individual liberty and privacy on the Y axis and control of pandemics on the X axis. We could then draw a line showing how the greater a society protects individual liberty and privacy, the less it can control germs in pandemics. MIT Media labs discovered that most apps used by foreign governments "expose the most private details about individuals."[21] As such, most Americans would view the apps as invasive. Of course, privacy is valued, or not valued, to different degrees around the world. In China, virtually no privacy exists: smart phones and cameras track the movements of every citizen. Facial recognition has advanced to such heights there that cameras recognize individual faces from a hundred feet away. With such surveillance, Chinese citizens who jaywalk or abandon rented bicycles in the wrong place are easily fined. If a Chinese citizen acquires enough demerits, he cannot fly or take a train. To travel anywhere after Covid, citizens of Wuhan had to download a color-oriented app on their phone, run by government computers. If they tried to leave Wuhan, police checked their phone and it had to show a Green Certificate. Thus, China made it easy for a contact tracer to identify and monitor infected Chinese people. If these infected or exposed citizens wanted to keep their privileges, they had to cooperate.[22]

When 3,000 passengers departed the Diamond Princess cruise ship in Taiwan, the government monitored infected passengers and their contacts by using data from credit cards, bus cards, and security cameras. They discovered 627,386 Taiwanese citizens who had been in the vicinity of an infected person and immediately texted them to urge them to be tested. Taiwan led the world in setting up convenient mass testing sites. South Korea and Iceland used similar phone apps and their citizens seemed fine with their governments knowing their every location and activity. Of course, such was not the case in the United States. For complex historical reasons, Americans value privacy, where the word is often a marker for personal liberty. For Americans, fundamental individual rights predate the state: Americans do not exist for the state, but the state exists to protect the rights of Americans to live their lives as they choose.

Cultural norms in Canada differed from those in the United States during the pandemic. Complaint lines, so-called "snitch lines," across Canada flooded authorities with tips about Canadians suspected of not wearing masks or not socially distancing, or of bars not enforcing government regulations. Facebook groups outed neighbors or suspicious individuals suspected of bringing the virus into communities. Canadians testing positive were often "Covid shamed," including a worker for the Canadian Broadcasting Corporation whose positive status forced him to re-locate across the country. In Nova Scotia, which had just 18 active cases in February 2021, one public health doctor lamented that "social media can be more virulent than the virus itself."[23]

Back in the United States, the great value put on individual rights and privacy defeated contact tracing. Americans during the Covid pandemic were deeply divided, with Trump supporters pitted against those against his policies. A survey in July 2019 by the Pew Research Center showed that 75 percent of Americans distrusted their government, and people who distrust government will not cooperate with contact tracers.[24] On the other hand, in countries with high satisfaction and happiness, such as Iceland, Denmark, and New Zealand, people gladly cooperated because if everyone already knows everyone else (Iceland), or sees the state as the source of benefits that bring happiness (Denmark), privacy is not a big concern.

All in all, the most basic assumption behind contact tracing is that the numbers of those infected are relatively small, and that if potentially infected citizens are contacted and encouraged to quarantine, the numbers of infections can be kept small. But what would happen if authorities were slow to start contact tracing and the number of infected persons was as high as 25 million? And given asymptomatic spread and many infected people with no or mild symptoms, those infected people might have had many contacts before learning they are infected. Therefore, in a country that allows widespread dissemination of the virus, contact tracing is largely ineffective.

By August 2020, then, many state and city leaders in the United States admitted that contact tracing had become a colossal failure. As the *New York Times* concluded then, "Contact tracing...has largely failed in the United States; the virus' pervasiveness and major lags in testing have rendered the system almost pointless. In some regions, large swaths of the population have refused to participate or cannot even be located, further hampering health care workers."[25]

PRIVACY OF GENETIC INFORMATION COLLECTED DURING TESTING IN PANDEMICS

One of the great issues in modern bioethics concerns the use of genetic information obtained by businesses and government agencies. Concerns about misuse of such information by insurance companies and employers led to the Genetic Information Nondiscrimination Act of 2008 (GINA), which forbids such entities from using genetic information about an individual to deny employment or coverage. Another important insight that modern bioethics has about such genetic information is that there is no such thing as testing only atomistic individuals. When George is tested for autosomal dominant genes such as those for Huntington's disease, George is also testing his parents and potentially giving them information (he cannot get the disease unless one of his parents has it). If Donna tests herself for the presence of one of the breast cancer genes and discovers she is positive, she is also learning something that may be true of her siblings, children, and parents.

Such knowledge can be useful in many ways. Genetic analysis has been crucial in finding serial killers who hid their identity for decades but who left semen or blood that could be analyzed. But the power of such analysis for law enforcement, as well as for amateur genealogists, depends on how many citizens put their genetic results on a public database. In this regard, the ongoing project of the National Institutes of Health, All of Us, is attempting to recruit one million Americans to be followed for life after having their genomes extensively mapped, with the hope that such mapping and cooperation will help scientists discover how the interplay of genetics, environments, and behavior prevents or causes various diseases. Advocates for genetic privacy, as well as the followers of Foucault and Agamben, worry that the state might use such information against Americans, posing yet another tradeoff between protecting individual rights and promoting the general welfare.

In this context, important questions must be asked about what happens to swabs tested for SARS2 and its variants. Good things can happen if stored samples are used correctly. In the 1980s, gay men in California donated blood samples to see if a vaccine worked against hepatitis B. The vaccine succeeded, and the samples were preserved. When HIV hit and irrational ideas circulated about who got infected and why, it was possible to use the same samples to prove that HIV was transmitted in the three ways we now know. In the same way, a study using donated blood of nuns in Florida showed that mosquitoes there did not transmit HIV (many HIV+ patients lived near the nuns, nuns got bitten often, but none were HIV+).

Might stored swabs with DNA of the millions tested for SARS2 be used in similarly beneficial ways? It might be possible to identify who is most likely to get sick, to die, or to be super-spreaders, and to make appropriate interventions. Advocates for privacy worry, though, that the same genetic analysis might stigmatize someone as a possible super-spreader and thus harm that person. Others worry that companies might use genetic information to hire only those workers who are unlikely to get sick and avoid those who are likely to get sick. On the dark side, what if personalized medicine reveals that those inheriting, say, allele X, are likely to be super-spreaders? Will they face discrimination in the workplace? What if general analysis reveals that those with the Z allele will likely die if put on a ventilator in the ICU? Will that information be used to deny them, in triage cases, access to ventilators? Will a different outcome, say, that allele BB gives them great prospects for recovery, privilege those people for ventilators or ICU beds? This is eerily reminiscent of a theme in the 1997 movie *Gattaca*, where society uses genetic information in fatalistic ways, dooming some people before they get a chance to try. Perhaps the future will allow genotyping into four groups: (1) those most likely to create massive antibodies to coronaviruses from vaccines, and hence who should be front-line workers, (2) those least likely to create massive antibodies to coronaviruses from vaccines, and hence those who should work from home, and (3) those most likely to die, or (4) not to die, from getting a coronavirus?

This might be true in the United States today, in companies that have policies for medical coverage where, if too many employees need very expensive treatment, premiums for all can be raised. For example, a very expensive treatment exists for the Hepatitis C virus. At the same time, white women have the IL28B genetic variant, which, after childbirth, helps their bodies clear the virus, but this variant is less frequent in people of African descent.[26] Some researchers have suggested rationing expensive treatment for Hepatitis C by this IL28B genotype, treating only those most at risk of not clearing the virus. Others have raised red flags about using genetic analysis for such triage decisions.

Parents in New York City wanted assurances from Fulgent Genetics, which collected swabs from their children for SARS2 analysis, that the samples would be destroyed after testing, which Fulgent said it would do. However, it does not appear that any law in New York or GINA requires Fulgent to do so.[27] Followers of Foucault and Agamben worry about the potential of the wrong entities to use such information against Americans, posing a risk to individual rights and privacy.

FURTHER READING

Agamben, Giorgio. *Homo Sacer: Sovereign Power and Bare Life*. Translated by Daniel Heller-Roazen. Stanford, CA: Stanford University Press, 1998.

Brizuela, Israel. *The Social and Privacy Impact of Contact Tracing for COVID-19: Strategies of COVID-19 in the Philippine Setting*. Amazon, 2020.

Foucault, Michel. *Power and Knowledge: Selected Interviews and Other Writings, 1972–1977*. Translated by Colin Gordon et al. New York: Vintage Books, 1980.

Kahn, Jeffrey, ed. *Digital Contact Tracing for Pandemic Response: Ethics and Governance Guidance*. Baltimore, MD: Johns Hopkins University Press, 2020.

CHAPTER 10
STATUS CERTIFICATES

Almost as soon as countries locked down and people avoided travel, others revived the idea of immunity passports, documents that would certify that the bearer previously had been exposed to a germ, had developed sufficient antibodies against it, or had been vaccinated. In early 2021, Israel required such a passport to clear citizens wanting to enter gyms, hotels, and some restaurants. Almost as soon as vaccination became a reality, some international airlines wanted to add Covid vaccinations to the standard vaccination cards used for international travel. An idea different from an immunity passport or vaccination certificate is a negative SARS2 test. This would be a PCR test that proves a person no longer has any SARS2 virus in their body. This chapter discusses such tests, passports, and cards and the ethical issues they raise.

DEFINING KEY TERMS

Several different kinds of documentation mentioned above are frequently confused. Let's begin with "immunity passport."

The first thing to notice is that a passport does not admit of degrees of immunity: either you have immunity or you don't. A passport allows you to enter and leave a country (there is no partial entry). On the other hand, the relative level of one's immunity is a matter of degrees, and what is measured here—antibodies from previous exposure to a virus—admits of variable degrees. It is crucial to next ask, "immunity from what?" If Anna is exposed to the original coronavirus from Wuhan, she will have very specific antibodies to that virus; now suppose she is issued an immunity certificate against SARS2. What does that guarantee? It is not clear that she is immune from infection from variants of SARS2, and more importantly, there are some documented cases of reinfection by SARS2. If Anna became reinfected and possessed a status certificate, yet worked as a bus driver or bartender, she could become a super-spreader. Next, we know that immunity from antibodies varies among people of different age groups and that it lessens over time. This is also true for immunity created from vaccinations, which may confer immunity for those over 70 for only 6 months, but for 12 months for those age 35.[1] We will explore this more below, but for now, these facts mean that any immunity certificate will need a time stamp to show when it expires. At this stage, though, such an expiration date would be extremely difficult to establish with certainty.

Next consider vaccination certificates, which will now probably be on smartphones. As previously explained, the goal of the clinical trials for both the Pfizer and Moderna vaccines was to prove a lack of major symptoms of Covid (fever, loss of smell and taste, etc.), but the goal was not to prove the absence of the coronavirus. The thousands of volunteers were not brought back and given a PCR test to show presence or absence of live virus in the body, so there is no proof that vaccination shows that the bearer of a vaccination certificate does not carry the coronavirus and, more important, that if they do, they cannot spread it to others. In the language of immunology, the Pfizer and Moderna vaccines were not designed to provide *sterilizing immunity*, which is complete absence of the virus in a person's body or in a population. The vaccine against measles, which SARS2 may resemble, gives sterilizing immunity, and vaccines that gave sterilizing immunity were the key to erasing the smallpox virus from the globe. Many vaccines used today—for example, the hepatitis B vaccine—do not provide sterilizing immunity. As pathology professor Dawn Bowdish of McMaster University explains, "A lack of sterilizing immunity means that the pathogen can continue to circulate in a population, where it may cause illness in unvaccinated and vulnerable people or evolve to evade our immune responses."[2]

Finally consider a negative SARS2 test, and for our purposes here, let's assume it's the gold standard and a PCR test. For the moment, let's put aside worries about false negatives and ask, "What does such a negative test show?" The answer is that it shows that the person tested did not have the virus *at the time he or she was tested*. If Anna is tested a week before she flies to Hawaii, it shows she wasn't infected a week ago, but it doesn't prove she didn't get infected during the following week or for that matter, during her flight.

In sum, "passport" is misleading because it does not admit of degrees. To say being vaccinated or having Covid gives one immunity is begging the question, because we don't know that vaccines make you immune against getting the virus at all (or getting a variant), and we don't know that getting sick once gives you permanent immunity from getting sick again, so "immunity certificate" is inaccurate. Finally, vaccination certificates differ from negative PCR tests, which prove only that you were negative at the time the test was given.

So what should we call all these kinds of documents? For convenience in this chapter, I will refer to all these documents as "status certificates," implying that a good status certificate could show prior infection, vaccination, repeated negative PCR tests for SARS2, or all of the above.

WHAT IS THE PURPOSE OF STATUS CERTIFICATES?

As explained, Covid vaccines weren't developed to prove that vaccinated people can't harbor the SARS2 virus or pass it on to others. "It's possible that someone could get the vaccine but could still be an asymptomatic carrier," said CNN medical analyst Dr. Leana Wen, an emergency physician. "They may not show symptoms, but they have the virus in their nasal passageway so that if they're speaking, breathing, sneezing and so on, they can still transmit it to others."[3] Here we also must distinguish between two different purposes of status certificates: protection of individuals versus protection of communities. For example, a status certificate could assure us that Rachel could work in a nursing home without getting Covid, but it would not guarantee that she couldn't spread SARS2 from one client to another. This would be especially true if, because of such a status certificate, Rachel was less diligent in using PPE than before getting such a certificate.

We also need to follow infectious disease classifications and distinguish between *natural immunity* after infection and *vaccine-induced immunity*.[1] At the start of 2021, the coronavirus and vaccines against it had not existed long enough for scientists to answer the following questions: (1) Do these immunities differ? (2) Do these immunities wane over time? (3) Does the lessening of immunity over time differ in the two kinds of immunity? Until scientists know the answers to these three questions, it will be hard to issue one all-encompassing status certificate for any long period of time.

Why don't we know more? In 2020, a study had been planned by the Covid-19 Prevention Network formed by the National Institute of Allergy and Infectious Diseases (NAID), headed by Anthony Fauci, that would follow 20,000 college students to see not only if the Moderna vaccine protected students against Covid but also if it prevented the virus from spreading person-to-person and whether it prevented infections that don't cause symptoms. Researchers, led by Larry Corey of Seattle's Fred Hutchinson Center, hoped to get all the 20,000 students nationwide vaccinated early in the spring semester of 2021 and then test them later to see if the vaccine met the other goals. Unfortunately, the study—which would have cost hundreds of millions of dollars—was not funded by the Trump administration for reasons that are unclear.[5] People speculated that its not being funded was due to the disarray of the last months of the Trump administration, but it's also possible that, given the problems in vaccine rollouts, students couldn't be vaccinated quickly enough before the end of spring term, and campus officials were already too overwhelmed monitoring and quarantining students to participate in a funded clinical trial.

In February 2021, Brazil started a three-month study with CoronaVac, the Chinese vaccine made by Sinovac, to discover whether those vaccinated against Covid can still transmit the virus.[6] All 45,000 residents of the town of Serrana in the São Paulo area will be vaccinated and followed. Dubbed "Project S," the study was kept secret to prevent thousands traveling to the town to get the vaccine. This study is highly relevant to status certificates because, without evidence that vaccines provide *sterilizing immunity*, all that a status certificate will accomplish is to prove that a vaccinated individual may work or travel in areas of infection without developing serious illness. However, there is still no guarantee that the same person will not spread the virus or its variants to others. A physician reported in early 2021 that she had seen "nearly 10 patients who got infected 10 days after the first dose [of a vaccine,] and 3 who got infected 2 weeks after the second dose."[7]

Recall that preliminary data for the clinical trial for the Moderna vaccine showed that the vaccine reduced viral transmission in two thirds of the volunteers, but possibly did not in the other third. Even this result is open to question: "As of today [January 12, 2021], there really is very little information" about viral transmission in vaccinated people, said researcher Larry Corey.[8] Now someone might object here, "But vaccines will prevent old people from getting sick or dying, and for young people, who often don't have severe symptoms, they will strengthen their immune systems, so they can do what they want." Isn't that true? The answer is: "It depends." If you are living with a kidney transplant, or must take immune-suppressing drugs, you don't want to interact with a health-care worker who's been vaccinated but still carrying a coronavirus. For such people, avoiding virus-carrying workers may be a life-or-death issue. This also means that hospitals and doctor's offices will need to be careful about who they hire and why.

The question of this section was "What is the purpose of status certificates?" But we could just as easily have asked, "Who are status certificates for?" One possibility is that they are for the bearer, whom we will call Ralph, to prove to him that he can interact with others and not fear getting sick or dying from a coronavirus. Another possibility is that status certificates would be intended for those around Ralph, so that they can interact with him and not fear getting sick. In that case, we would want a high degree of certainty that vaccinated Ralph or post-Covid Ralph can't transmit a coronavirus. Yet another possibility is that status certificates are for those who might employ Ralph, so they can be assured they will not get sued by other workers because Ralph infected them. This may be a big deal, because workplace lawsuits about Covid skyrocketed in 2020.[9]

BENEFITS OF STATUS CERTIFICATES

As an official piece of documentation, status certificates could be important tools, allowing people to resume living normal lives and regain the benefits of free movement in a modern society, such as the ability to fly safely or to eat in a public restaurant.

Let's give one scenario some rope and see if it hangs itself. Let's assume that the tests behind a status certificate are completely accurate. Let's also assume that people with status certificates must wear a biometric device like a Fitbit that monitors their antibodies to SARS2. Let's assume, too, that when a person loses Covid antibodies, or doesn't have enough of them, their certificate switches from green to red. Let's assume further that once a person has been infected and has antibodies, they cannot pass on the virus to someone else or get reinfected. In sum and for the moment, set aside worries about the problems of the accuracy of status certificates and assume that they can actually prove that those who hold them are safe for others to be around. Call them good status certificates. Under these assumptions, it is obvious that if everyone working at Sam's Grocery has a status certificate, it's safer for everyone working there, and for everyone shopping there, than if the viral status of everyone were unknown. Likewise, for two athletic teams about to engage in a physical contest, it's safer for everyone if all athletes have status certificates. The same goes for weddings, funerals, concerts, conventions, and marathons. In general, accurate status certificates could make social life safer for everyone in the way driver's licenses do.

Good status certificates point a way for many businesses to re-open safely. Such certificates could rejuvenate international travel. For Mexico, the United States, and Canada, air travel matters a lot. Air travel, and the tourist industries it supports, is a multi-billion-dollar industry. Whole states and countries, such as Hawaii and Iceland, have economies that depend on tourists arriving by airplane. Canada and the United States have major cities on both east and west coasts, making it essential that businesspeople and families be able to easily get back and forth. But without the mythically perfect Covid document described above, how do countries resume normal business travel and tourism?

In 2020, airports and airlines tried to facilitate safe travel by not only requiring passengers to wear masks but also offering testing to ensure that all passengers on board had tested negative within 48 to 72 hours before their flight.[10] That testing was cumbersome and time-consuming. Passengers could fly to Alaska, get a $250 test, but then had to isolate for a few days while awaiting results. The ideas of waiting in a hotel room for a few days to see when, and if, your Alaskan vacation could begin did not appeal to many people. The same thing with flying to Thailand and awaiting your results from a lab inside the Bangkok airport, where if negative you were cleared to leave but if positive you were taken to a Thai hospital.

Rapid tests offer a better solution. Already on international flights, passengers must check in at least an hour before take-off or lose their seats. All flights now require passengers to wear masks; they may soon require passengers to be SARS2-free before boarding. Flight attendants and pilots would certainly endorse that policy, as well as gate agents, baggage handlers, and other airport staff. In 2021, the European Union was developing a "digital green pass" for EU citizens, which would show vaccination status and/or results of SARS2 tests. Airlines and countries dependent on international tourism were also pushing versions of status certificates, especially for use on smartphones. But can we require passengers to have a status certificate before flying? Of course. No one has a right to fly sick with an infectious disease. For most people, flying on planes is a public outing and, as such, people can harm each other by their bad behavior, making their actions on such planes into moral issues. In 2020, nearly 2,500 flight attendants became infected with SARS2, prompting the Biden administration in 2021 to mandate wearing masks on planes.[11]

In developed countries, the service industry makes up a third or more of jobs, covering workers in restaurants, bars, gyms, theme parks, interior design, and renovation, as well as service personnel who fix problems in residences. Knowing such workers have status certificates would allow prospective customers to feel safe around them again. Therefore, an important argument for ideal status certificates is economic. Tourism supports the economies of many places such as New Orleans, Hawaii, Florida, Thailand, and Cape Town, as well as the economies of cruise ships. Tourists will not return in previous numbers until they feel safe, and that will require not mere rhetoric and manipulation but evidence. Many tourists with the most money and leisure are seniors, but they are also more vulnerable to Covid and will resist traveling until they feel safe. Good status certificates will allow that.

Good status certificates could also help first responders. Knowing who's likely to be infected matters to those who treat strangers every day in emergencies. Good status certificates could also help daycare centers, nursing homes, group homes, and prisons find staff to work there, staff who don't fear getting Covid and who are increasingly hard to find.

In the early 1980s, earnest hospital administrators urged staff to treat every patient "as if" they were HIV+ to create maximal safety for all, and for a while that was done, but if only 0.1 percent of your patients are HIV+, it wastes time and equipment to treat every patient that way. Over time, tests that rapidly identified HIV allowed staff to take extra precautions for HIV-infected patients only. If EMT responders could also separate those who are not at risk for Covid from those who are, this would make their lives safer. This is especially important if someone had a heart attack and needed CPR, where chest compressions spew aerosols into the air.

PROBLEMS WITH STATUS CERTIFICATES

Some critics fear that status certificates will discriminate against those who are infected or unvaccinated. The Canadian bioethicist Françoise Baylis has been especially vocal about the immorality of status certificates. Baylis, of Dalhousie University, and molecular biologist Natalie Kofler, of Harvard University, argue that status certificates are "ethically problematic" because they would (1) "exacerbate current inequities [and] . . . create a novel layer of biological inequity."[12] They think such certificates are unfeasible because (2) they would require too many tests, (3) they might encourage people to intentionally get infected to get a Green certificate, (4) there might not be enough workers cleared with Green certificates to help the economy, and (5) they would harm people from poor nations who are unable to get them.

Let's consider these arguments. The idea that people will intentionally get infected to get a status certificate seems silly or reckless, at least in many places. With so much of the virus around, Sam doesn't need to deliberately infect himself because if he acts irresponsibly long enough, he will get infected. It was for this reason that human challenge studies were unnecessary: so much virus was around that those in both treatment and placebo groups quickly got exposed. The objection that status certificates would require too many tests also seems inadequate because it assumes that we will always have expensive, delayed testing. That will change. For example, Germany in 2021 approved a rapid PCR test for SARS2 that used only a book-sized box and gave results, not as previous PCR tests produced in 2–3 days, but in 40 minutes.[13] This is the same country that developed the first test for SARS2—the one adopted by the WHO and not the United States—and that supported the NBiotech company, which partnered with Moderna for the second successful vaccine. At its approval, the test was 90-percent accurate and almost as good as lab-based PCR tests. More important, the National Institutes of Health is spending $1 billion in its RADX program to develop fast, easy-to-use, and accessible testing for SARS2.[14] With that kind of money pushing them, good, rapid tests will soon be here.

The objection that there might not be enough workers with status certificates to help the economy also seems incorrect. As we've seen, workers could get such a certificate in three ways: vaccination, prior infection, or negative PCR test. With millions getting vaccinated every week, there should be enough workers to help the economy, and besides, many workers were required to work, for example in construction, during the pandemic without a status certificate, so what about them? Why wouldn't this continue indefinitely? Just because some employers might require status certificates doesn't mean most would. This objection seems not to be a strong one.

As for the objection that status certificates for Canadians and Americans would hurt people from poor nations unable to get them, well, that is true for almost any innovation, whether it's the first smartphones, the Internet, PReP to prevent HIV, substitution medication for addiction, or assisted reproduction. The acts-and-omissions doctrine enters here: not giving money to save starving people in Somalia differs from sending such people poisoned food. Giving your teenagers smartphones may make Somali teenagers jealous, but it doesn't harm them.

This leaves us with the ethical objection that status certificates will increase social and economic inequality, and it is to that objection that we now turn.

A New Caste System?

Françoise Baylis's worries that status certificates would be used by elitists to exclude Covid-infected or Covid-exposed people seemed to be realized at swanky parties in the Hamptons on Long Island, New York, in 2020, where private for-hire physicians offered quick testing to guests in limousines who waited for negative results before entering the host's estate.[15] The private service used a Quidel testing machine and charged $500 a test. Access to such testing may soon become a mark of high status. As Mary Ann Mackey of Brooklyn's Park Slope, who waited hours for her results at another party on the first weekend in August 2020, remarked, "This feels like a weird thing to say, but it was kind of a cool experience. It felt like a privilege to have results."[16] Similarly, Knightsbridge Circle in London, a club charging £25,000 a year for membership, offered members flights to the United Arab Emirates, where they could vacation for three weeks and receive the first and second doses of the Pfizer vaccine. After the club made the offer, it received more than 2,000 new applications for membership.[17]

Cosmopolitans versus Nationalists

We saw in Chapter 7 that globalism competes today with nationalism in the ownership and distribution of vaccines, and we see the same tension between these two perspectives over status certificates. Globalists are often called "cosmopolitans" because they identify as citizens of the world and dislike national borders. As such, they seek to diminish the importance of borders as much as possible, making us all citizens of the world. Philosopher Kwame Anthony Appiah of New York University, who was born in Ghana and educated in England, and who writes the "Ethicist" column each week for the *New York Times Magazine*, has argued for this ideal in his *Cosmopolitanism: Ethics in a World of Strangers*.[18] Cosmopolitans would move us toward fewer distinctions between the people of the earth and toward more equality. As such, cosmopolitans oppose status certificates as creating another distinction between people and decreasing the economic opportunities available to people to move freely across borders. For cosmopolitans, a status certificate is like Britain pulling out of the European Union, making a distinction between people where previously there wasn't one.

But cosmopolitanism has its critics. As long as some countries provide better benefits and generally provide better lives for immigrants and their children, families will leave failed countries for countries where they can live better. The late biologist Garrett Hardin criticized the open-borders approach as analogous to a letting everyone into a lifeboat after a shipping disaster.[19] The boat, or a country, he argued, just doesn't have enough resources to support everyone who wants to enter. Imagine if a small British town allowed all of its farmers to graze their cows at will on town commons grasslands. Eventually, overgrazing and destruction of the commons would occur (hence Hardin's name for this problem—the *tragedy of the commons*).

The Essential Objection to Status Certificates

The fundamental ethical objection to status certificates has so far not been well described in this book. For many critics of such certificates, that objection boils down to a fear that such certificates will intensify existing inequality. In her address to the Nuffield Council of Ethics, an organization that has made important contributions to bioethics in the United Kingdom and worldwide, Bobbie Farsides, who has taught since 2006 at Brighton and Sussex Medical School as Professor of Clinical and Biomedical Ethics, sketches how the pandemic has harmed BAME (Black, Asian, and Minority Ethnic) communities in Britain.[20] She notes with approval that some homeless and disabled people, unable to physically distance in congregate housing, got special housing during the pandemic—housing which might be taken away if they got status certificates that allowed them to live anywhere. But she notes with disapproval the attack by fiscal conservatives on the National Health System and the government of Boris Johnson's emphasis on protecting the economy rather than protecting the most vulnerable: "It is against this background that we must ask whether the immunity certificate is the correct means to an end we feel safe for our government to prioritize and pursue?"[21]

Clearly, she does not trust the Johnson government's approach because "immunity certification is primarily a ticket back into the marketplace—a means of exercising your negative liberty" ("negative liberty" is the right to be left alone to pursue your goals). Clearly, she is not interested in such a marketplace—small business owners and unemployed workers—and instead urges the government to foster "feelings of solidarity, common purpose and collaboration." Given the hard feelings caused by Brexit, finalized at the end of 2020, she fears that status certificates would amplify the existing sense of "us" versus "them," especially when the system "categorized people in terms of their relationship to a virus and treated them accordingly."[22]

This view is echoed by Alexandra Phelan, an assistant professor of microbiology at Georgetown University whose research focuses on infectious diseases and global security. Like Farsides, Phelan believes that status certificates might alleviate the "duty of governments to adopt policies that protect economic, housing, and health rights." She believes that such certificates "would be ripe for corruption and implicit bias" ("implicit bias" describes negative attitudes towards groups of people that we might have without conscious awareness). She also believes that traditional vaccination cards incentivize for social goods (protecting others from infection), while status certificates in contrast "incentivize infection."[23]

Against this kind of view, bioethicist Julian Savulescu and colleagues at Oxford University's Uehiro Centre for Practical Ethics argued in 2020 that if its effect on existing inequality was the sole judge of whether an innovation should be introduced to society, virtually nothing would pass.[24] They also argue that the presumption in a democracy must be personal freedom to travel, work, and form associations, and that because status certificates further those freedoms, the onus of proof is on anyone who would deny them. Because lockdowns might exist for a long time, or during future pandemics, anything that allowed a proportion of the population during those periods to access more freedoms would be a good thing. They conclude: "The choice is not between returning to a normal life versus issuing immunity passports. Instead, the choice is between periodic lockdowns, attempting to emerge from lockdowns with immunity passports, and attempting to emerge from lockdowns without immunity passports. Immunity passports are a potentially valuable and ethical tool."[25]

Finally, one might argue that it's not going to be *vaccine certificates* that increase inequality between rich and poor but the *vaccinations themselves* that do so. If vaccine inequality grows, the world may soon see a gap between those securely vaccinated and those who are not, between those who can live and travel safely and those who cannot, and between those who can safely work closely together and those who cannot. If vaccines are required yearly against new variations, such a gap may only increase.

A License to Party?

If status certificates bring about any intended behaviors, it will likely not be by people throwing "Covid parties" to get infected (probably an urban legend),[26] but by people who misinterpret status certificates themselves. Some people misinterpret vaccination and think of it as a "Get Out of Jail Free" card, such that immediately after vaccination they throw off their masks, stop physical distancing, and join large groups.

What they don't know is that, first, most vaccines take a week to ten days to create antibodies; second, the first dose of two-dose vaccines just starts the process of creating antibodies; third, after three weeks with only one dose, those antibodies can start to wane if not followed by a second dose; and fourth, after the second dose, it takes another week to ten days to mount a full antibody response. Because some of those vaccinated may feel invulnerable, they may not realize that people who have been vaccinated can get infected after their shots.[27] As the CDC says, building immunity "typically takes a few weeks...that means it's possible a person could be infected with the virus that causes COVID-19 just before or just after vaccination and still get sick."[28] Preliminary data from Israel showed that 70 percent of Israelis who got the Pfizer vaccine could still get infected after the first shot.[29]

An example of how status certificates could easily lead to breakdowns in public health occurred in one of the first good studies published in 2021 of infection after an 18-hour airplane trip of 86 passengers from Dubai to New Zealand, which has a zero-tolerance policy for SARS2, requires a 14-day quarantine period at mandated hotels, and rigorously tests any new arrivals during these two weeks. Even though the plane was only one-quarter full (it could carry 400 passengers), New Zealand discovered that seven of the passengers eventually tested positive and four became infected during the flight.[30] The crucial issue is that five of those seven passengers had taken a test for SARS2 in the days before the flight and tested negative, but Patient Zero (the source of the infection for the other four) had tested negative even earlier: a full five days before the flight. And on the flight, the airline operated on the opposite of the Swiss Cheese Model: rather than having multiple layers of protection—mandatory wearing of masks throughout the trip, distancing of six feet or more in all directions, and requiring passengers not to mingle—the airline relied too much on the apparent lack of symptoms, voluntary behavior, and the above-mentioned tests. Obviously, accepting a negative test five days before the flight was a mistake.

Are the Tests Accurate?

The physician in charge of disease control for the state of New York warned would-be party-goers in the Hamptons that their results before their swanky party could be unreliable: "A negative test does not preclude one not to be carrying the virus," he said.[31] This is true because, first of all, SARS2 may not be detectable in the body by any test for as long as ten days, which is why, after being exposed to a person with the virus, this is usually the minimal time of quarantine. Second, the accuracy of results depends on what kind of test has been used. A PCR test for the presence of the virus is more accurate than a test for antibodies. A good viral test should be able to distinguish between testing for live virus versus particles of dead virus. (Because they retain particles of dead virus, do some people test positive for months after infection? We are unsure.) Third, a test for antibodies to the virus is even more problematic. One of the most basic questions concerns how long immunity lasts after infection. Anthony Fauci says, "The antibody response traditionally in coronaviruses in general is nothing like measles, which lasts essentially for life. It isn't even in the same ballpark. We had a bunch of papers to show that it has a relatively short duration of 6 months to a year or so."[32]

Exactly how many antibodies should one have, and at what age should one get a status certificate? Do antibodies vary with severity of first infection? And are some antibodies, for various reasons, more effective than others? A study of 12,000 health-care workers at Oxford University Hospitals published in 2021 found that the presence of anti-spike or anti-nucleocapsid IgC antibodies prevented both symptomatic and asymptomatic infection by SARS2 (confirmed by PCR tests) for six months.[33] But what about nine months later? A year? Studies also need to be done about the rate of false negatives and false positives. No test is perfect, and people differ in their physiology and blood types, skewing reactions to some tests. Nor do children always test the same way as adults. All these things need to be studied and known before status certificates become the gold standard of post-pandemic life.

Most important of all, against which strains has a person been vaccinated or tested? If only the original strain, then those possessing such certificates could be potentially traveling freely around carrying a document clearing them for only one of many variants—rendering the certificate useless in preventing the spread of SARS2. We already know that B117, P1, and B1351 have been spreading around the world and we know that other variants emerged in California, New York, and Oregon. Does a negative certificate for the original strain of SARS2 guarantee that the bearer has not been exposed (or does not carry) any of the variants, especially variants with the Eek mutation that seem to evade the body's immune system?

Other Problems

Given such misinterpretations, one wonders how status certificates will be used, or misused, with relationships and dating apps. Will potential partners take status certificates as a guarantee of a person being clear of the virus and of the potential to pass it on? If so, what happens when potential partners become positive after dating? Bioethics covers a lot of ground and therefore raises a wide range of questions concerning how status certificates might be used or misused. Will they be needed for transplanted organs? Donated sperm or eggs? Entry into a nursing home? Acceptance to nursing or medical school?

And what about long-haulers? When those with Long Covid retain the virus for months after their initial infection, will they be denied status certificates? In these cases, the virus may reside within reservoirs of internal organs and be hard to root out. Long-haulers are probably not infectious but may test SARS2 positive on a PCR test. What about people who never showed symptoms but who keep testing positive by PCR tests? Presumably, neither group could get a status certificate.

Such certificates would also need a time stamp to cover the worst-case scenarios. As of early 2021, we think that SARS2 infections give those who are infected antibodies for at least six months.[34] If that is the minimum length, and if antibodies block viral infection and transmission, then immunity certificates would only be good for six months after infection. They would need to be renewed by testing every six months. If you have antibodies for one strain that last six months, then are infected with a new strain three months later, and another strain three months after that, you could have to be on a yearly, rolling renewal, hypothetically for as many times as there are variants.

Also, which vaccines will legitimate international travel? Will the Cuban, Chinese, and Russian vaccines count? China will accept only visitors who have had its vaccines. Most of the world (86 countries) will use the AstraZeneca vaccine, but it is not approved for use in the United States. What about just one dose of Pfizer or Moderna? What about people who have religious objections to any vaccines or specifically to vaccines in any way connected to fetal tissue? Can countries ban them from travel or entry into public buildings?

Some advocates for privacy fear that, like driver's licenses, status certificates could be used for other purposes, such as discovering undocumented workers and forcing them to leave a country (and if this is true, it would mean such workers would resist vaccination). In Britain, for this reason officials feared resistance to vaccination from undocumented people, so the wallet-sized vaccination card issued by the National Health Service did not list the person's name or any other personal information.[35]

Various groups tied to business and airlines are developing digital health passes (apps) for smartphones.[36] If airlines in Europe, Asia, and North America ever agree on who should pay for such apps and on how they should be used, they still seem designed for those who can afford both smartphones and international travel, thus exacerbating gaps of class and wealth. And what about fraud? If status certificates became valuable, what would nefarious people do to get one? By April 2021, one could easily buy forged vaccine certificates on the Internet,[37] and airlines struggled to detect falsified certificates on international flights.[38] Could someone who did not get vaccinated say he lost his vaccination card and request another? In Britain, doesn't the lack of a name or personal information open such cards up to fraud and fakes? Also, could someone who has antibodies offer their blood sample to someone else to help them get a certificate, like using someone else's urine to pass a drug test?

At present, states differ in how they issue vaccination certificates. In Washington state, for example, those vaccinated receive a card with their name, the name of the vaccine administered, and the date of each dosage. In Vermont, and probably to speed up the process, some of those vaccinated simply got a blank card. A bigger problem is that the United States lacks a national identity card that could be used to identify who is safe to fly. Nor does the country have an effective, national vaccine database that entities such as airlines and cruise ships might use to verify passenger vaccination.[39]

All this controversy allowed Florida's governor Ron DeSantis to ban Florida and its cities from issuing status certificates, and to prohibit public events from demanding them. In an unusual alliance, liberals championing privacy or who were worried about a vaccine-caste system hailed his ban, thus creating a wedge issue among both liberals and businesspeople.

FINAL NOTE

Although the main objections in bioethics to status certificates have stemmed from concerns about worsening inequality and hurting marginalized groups, these objections are weak compared to objections that hold that status certificates may give their bearers false assurances. Until we know with good evidence that a vaccinated person, a person with a certain number of antibodies, or a person with a proven prior infection cannot retain, or regain, a coronavirus and pass it to others, it is doubtful that status certificates can be used to normalize life. Worse, they could give their bearers a false sense of safety, making them stop the "Three Rules" of masking, distancing, and frequent hand washing, and contribute to the further spread of the virus.

In 2021, the Biden administration required a negative test for anyone (including Americans on returning flights) entering the United States, and five different kinds of tests were being accepted by early spring. A continuing problem for airlines and passengers was the lack of a consistent test, both inside the United States and Canada, as well as internationally.[40]

CHAPTER 11
STRUCTURAL INEQUALITIES AND VULNERABLE GROUPS

In an influential paper, Paul Farmer, a member of the Harvard medical faculty and noted for his Herculean efforts to help Haiti's poor, critiqued most bio-ethicists for focusing on problems of the well-off—on artificial hearts, assisted reproduction, intersex and gender, for example—while ignoring the problems of "those down below," who faced problems such as a lack of clean drinking water.[1]

What would make us more compassionate to "those down below"? One could imagine us all entering a Rawlsian social contract under a veil of ignorance about our personal position, race, gender, or medical coverage and asking how we would choose the basic structure of society, including medical coverage and testing/care during pandemics. One hopes this imaginary experiment would make us feel more compassionate for those at the bottom of society who become infected. But what if we don't live in a perfectly just society? Well, just as pandemics bring out the best and worst in individuals, in unjust societies they amplify the harms experienced by vulnerable people. This chapter explores how pandemics affect those who are most vulnerable.

WHO IS MOST VULNERABLE IN A PANDEMIC?

Prisoners may be the most vulnerable group during pandemics because as captives, they live in crowded conditions. In the United States, which incarcerates more citizens per capita than any nation in the world, at least one in five state and federal prisoners became infected with Covid in 2020, a total of at least 275,000, with at least 1,700 deaths. Because not all states recorded or released data about Covid-infected prisoners, these statistics are, according to one leading expert, "a vast undercount."[2] Kansas, for instance, had no plans to vaccinate its prisoners, and half became infected. Also, people of color constitute a disproportionate number of prisoners in the United States. Although liberal New York state planned to vaccinate guards and staff in its prisons, it had no plans to vaccinate its prisoners ahead of its citizens.[3] By July, San Quentin State Prison in California had more than a thousand infections.[4] And, although technically not prisoners, migrants trying to enter a country illegally are held in crowded detention centers and are highly vulnerable to infection. Although viruses don't distinguish between undocumented workers and legal citizens, when the Biden administration announced plans to vaccinate undocumented workers, its plan angered some legal citizens.

Under the Rawlsian conception of justice, all such groups should—at the minimum—*not be last* for testing, treatment, or resources. After all, being sent to jail for two years for theft (or possession of marijuana) should not be a death sentence, and likewise, living in a group home should not be the same. Residents of nursing homes ("care homes" in Britain) count as vulnerable, because they live and eat close together, often lack freedom of movement, and often have multiple medical problems. Because they had not committed crimes or tried to enter the country illegally, they got vaccinated early in the United States. Canada had major problems keeping those in its nursing homes safe or vaccinating them, resulting in many deaths.

Another vulnerable group comprises those who live in group homes for people with conditions such as autism, cerebral palsy, mental illness, and dementia. Similar homes support thousands of people who flee lives of prostitution, alcoholism, addiction, or spousal abuse. In addition, members of the Armed Forces living close together, in barracks, aircraft carriers, submarines, or military bases abroad may easily spread infections to one another and could be considered vulnerable. Cases on military bases mirrored infections in the country as a whole: on June 10, 2020, the military had 7,500 cases, but by July 20, that number had grown to 22,200 cases.[5]

When considering which essential workers are most vulnerable to infection or death, the list includes those who work in mass transit and meat-packing plants, migrant agricultural workers, soldiers on military bases and ships, and emergency responders. More police officers died of Covid in 2020 than from the

9/11 attacks on the World Trade Center.[6] As the economy pivoted to home delivery from Amazon and Walmart, workers in warehouses increasingly became infected and died. In many places in the United States, construction continued on building sites, exploiting the need to work of many male workers there. Under the Trump administration, the OSHA (Occupational Health and Safety Administration) did not investigate the prevalence of SARS2 in meat-packing plants, or of Covid deaths there, so the official figure of 239 Covid deaths and 45,000 infections is surely way too low.[7] The Biden administration promptly reversed this neglect, ordering new protections for such workers and new reporting requirements. Tyson Foods and Purdue Farms, for example, refused to test workers in their meat-packing plants, many of them recently arrived Americans living paycheck to paycheck.

Recall that we know that constant exposure to higher levels of coronavirus radically increases risks of infection, regardless of how much PPE medical staff wear, no matter how cautious they are. We know that, officially, at least 2,900 health-care workers died from Covid in 2020, but because the Trump administration resisted tracking any Covid deaths among such workers, the number is surely much higher, perhaps double.[8] Many states left out of their vaccination plans the nation's million-plus grocery workers, who were exposed daily to many customers, some of whom refused to wear masks. One remedy for workers in meatpacking plants, on assembly lines, and in grocery stores is to provide them N95 respirators, pump in fresh air from outside to dilute the virus, space workers six feet apart with plastic partitions, and if fresh air is not possible, install high-quality air filters. As Linsey Marr, the premier expert on airborne transmission in the United States, said, "It's time to stop pussyfooting around the fact that the virus is transmitted mostly through the air."[9]

Infections by Zip Code

Living in impoverished neighborhoods creates vulnerabilities to toxins and infectious agents. One study in 2019 analyzed health data by zip codes in the 500 largest US cities and found that life expectancy varied by as much as 30 years between neighborhoods in the same city.[10] On average, those in the more affluent zip codes in a city lived 20 years more than those in the least affluent neighborhoods of the same city. In big cities, well-off infected patients go to some hospitals and the least well-off infected go to others, with different levels of services, amenities, and staff. In New York City during its spring 2020 Covid surge, Mount Sinai Hospital's branch in the Bronx got many severely ill patients on Medicaid, whereas Cornell-Weill Hospital on the Upper East Side attended predominantly to patients with private insurance and had much better staffing and resources. Similar data explain why in many cities, people of color in poor neighborhoods get infected and die of Covid at much higher rates than people in middle-class, white neighborhoods. For example, the neighborhood of Gulfton in Houston, Texas, where 45,000 refugees, restaurant workers, immigrants, and poor people live, had nearly a thousand infections and 12 deaths, whereas in its middle-class suburb of Bellaire, home to mostly white and Asian professionals, only 67 people had been infected.[11]

Some injustices during pandemics are obvious, as when professional people can flee outbreaks in crowded cities to retreats in mountains, on seashores, or in rural cabins, avoiding exposure while working remotely and keeping families close. Other injustices concern lack of coverage for basic medical care, which affects seeking testing. If you don't know how to get a test, you don't know exactly what's wrong with you. Once you do know, you need to be sure that entering a hospital won't lead to your being deported. If you must quarantine to prevent infecting others, ideally you should confine yourself in a separate room, an option that many low-income individuals lack. If your children get exposed or infected and must attend school remotely, they need Internet access and computer equipment. If your job forces you to leave young children alone at home, someone must, ideally, attend to them, should they need help or get into trouble.

For those living in poor zip codes, one remedy is to offer vaccinations there, especially where residents lack access to mass transportation. Traveling buses or vans can visit rural towns; indeed, some states activated the National Guard to do this. And what if you have no zip code but are still vulnerable? The hundreds of thousands of foreign workers trapped offshore on cruise ships, some of whom were held there for six months, received little help or compassion, as was the case on ships that were unable to unload their crews anywhere in the fourteenth century because locals feared infection.[12] Such foreign workers being held offshore raises a difficult ethical problem about who is responsible for them.

Is Vaccination by Age Unjust?

One question that is rarely raised concerns why citizens over age 65 should automatically get vaccinated ahead of members of many vulnerable groups and essential workers. Medicare covers US citizens over age 65 and in 2020 covered 44 million Americans. A good percentage of them are neither medically fragile nor working in at-risk occupations. So why should healthy retirees in Florida or Arizona get vaccinated before grocery workers, prisoners, or teachers? Is it because such citizens vote in large percentages and regularly, having disproportionate political clout?

The city of Long Beach, California, offers a different model. After vaccinating medical staff and residents of nursing homes, it vaccinated grocery-store workers, teachers, and school staff, and because California made it do so, also those over age 65.[13] By vaccinating people this way, Long Beach at least made overlooked groups feel they weren't expendable, the way they felt in other states.[14]

Nevertheless, most states and countries slowly opened vaccinations by age from most elderly to age 16. States such as Florida that targeted nursing homes saw deaths and hospitalizations drop among the elderly. "The people who die [of Covid] tend to be older," said Ashish Jah, dean of Brown's School of Public Health, "and we've vaccinated a lot of people over 55 now [as of March 28, 2021]."[15]

African American, Latinx, and Covid

African Americans and Latinx became infected with SARS2 and died of Covid at higher rates than white Americans.[16] In Alabama, where African Americans make up about a quarter of the state's population, they accounted for nearly half of Covid deaths.[17] These facts raise two questions: Why did this happen? and What should be done about it? As we saw in the first chapters, throughout history, when epidemics and pandemics hit, victims have been blamed. Sometimes bigots claim a group's free, irresponsible behavior brought on their illness, so they deserved what they got. For example, the Irish historically have been blamed for problems caused by drinking. But attributing responsibility for illness is very tricky and often falsely judgmental. So we don't want to claim that some behavior of African Americans brought Covid upon them.

What could be called "crypto blaming" can also occur, in other words, using obesity and its related medical conditions as indirect ways of blaming victims for dying of Covid. Consider the following facts about Covid and obesity. First, two special categories in medicine are "obese," defined as having a BMI (Body Mass Index) over 30, and "severe obesity" (BMI over 40), and patients defined in these ways are at increased risk to experience heart problems, diabetes, mobility issues, and stroke. It is sometimes difficult to secure a large bed for severely obese patients or to place those patients in a prone position to enhance their respiration. Second, obese, SARS2-infected people were twice as likely to be hospitalized and, once there, 50-percent more likely to die of Covid.[18] In the CDC's study of 150,000 patients hospitalized for Covid, 77 percent were obese or severely obese, an alarming fact for the 42 percent of Americans classified as obese.[19]

A third fact related to obesity is that many people believe that obese individuals are responsible for their weight and, if they really tried, could lose it and maintain normal weight.[20] A final fact is that African-American, Latinx, First Peoples, Māori, and Hawaiian members of poorer communities represent a disproportionate percentage of obese people. Thus, people who are obese are both more likely to die from Covid and are more likely to be people of color. If one assumes that a relatively high percentage of middle-aged people of color are overweight and have chronic medical problems, does that make them responsible for being more likely to become infected with SARS2 or more likely to die from Covid? A more probable explanation for why Latinx and African Americans had higher rates of infection is that they worked in jobs where they were regularly exposed to lots of virus. Bus drivers, workers in meat-packing plants, first responders, aides in nursing homes, and cashiers in grocery stores were constantly exposed to infected, asymptomatic carriers.

People of color are also much more likely to live in cramped quarters with mixed or multi-generational families where the virus can spread easily. People of color are much more likely to live in segregated neighborhoods where they are more likely to be in contact with infected people. People of color are more likely to live in areas with poor public transportation and lack personal cars. People of color are more likely to lack medical or dental insurance. People of color are more likely not to have adequate living quarters to use to quarantine a member of their family exposed to SARS2 or sick with Covid. One of the most plausible explanations for the high rates of infection and death from Covid for people of color is that they are much more likely to work in jobs where they lack social distancing, where they are exposed to the virus in intense concentrations, and where they are exposed many times—people such as aides in day care, cafeteria workers and housekeepers in schools, and bus drivers.[21] For Native Americans, who may have several generations living together in cramped quarters, the virus quickly spread among family members. In Mississippi, almost 10 percent of the Choctaw tribe's 11,000 members were infected by August 2020, and 75 had died.[22] On the Navajo Indian reservations in New Mexico and Arizona and the trailers inhabited by migrant workers in Florida, three generations may live in two rooms.

The reasons that people of color and Indigenous peoples in North America arrived at this state are well known, complex, and beyond the scope of this book to describe. But given the legacy of slavery in North and South America, as well as the terrible toll of previous pandemics on the First Peoples of the Americas, the reasons that so many are still marginalized are not difficult to understand.[23] There is also an additional explanation as to why people of color are more vulnerable to Covid. As noted in Chapter 3, some people develop severe Covid because they have "enhanced IL-1-beta responses" or "perforin pathway mutations," which may cause cytokine storm syndrome. About 40 percent of African Americans inherit genetic polymorphisms associated with enhanced IL-1 production, but only 6 percent of Caucasians do. This may help explain why African Americans, when infected with SARS2, die of Covid more often.[24]

So many factors explain why disproportionate numbers of people of color die of Covid, most beyond their control. Even when people have some control over their weight, smoking, drinking, or addictions, when they get sick, we don't deny them care, and (for the most part) we don't blame them. Given the disproportionate numbers of deaths, what can be done to move a society further toward justice? Lacking a magic wand to change structural inequalities, advocates for people of color have focused on three things: free testing, free care, and priority for vaccinations. The first two objectives were attained in the United States and Canada: testing is free for everyone and the CARES Act reimburses American hospitals for medical treatment of all patients, regardless of their insurance status. This often has to be explained to undocumented workers who fear high medical bills or deportation if they enter hospitals as Covid patients for treatment.[25] Many Latinx workers in southern California, for example, did not know that Covid-testing was free and that they were entitled to paid sick leave.[26] We turn now to the third objective of advocates for people of color: vaccination priority.

Priority for Vaccination?

Various advocates for people of color have urged authorities to vaccinate African Americans first or early, explicitly by ranking them with front-line medical workers or by taking vaccines door-to-door in African-American neighborhoods.[27] *New York Times* columnist Ross Douthat argued this way, almost implying that not to do so was unjust.[28]

This plan has three big problems. First, whenever there is distribution of a benefit to a specific racial group—be it admissions to elite colleges, to medical school, or an organ transplant—other groups will see it as unjust and racist. On the face of it, it seems to violate the Kantian maxim of treating everyone the same and equally. And who counts as belonging to such groups. If it's Black Americans, how "Black" do you need to be to qualify? Will 25 percent count? One-eighth? In applying to medical schools or colleges, many universities allow applicants to self-identify their race or ethnicity. Would that work for priority to vaccination? Second, how do you explain why one vulnerable group gets vaccinated before another vulnerable group? What about disadvantaged Asians in San Francisco, Navajo on reservations in New Mexico, all prisoners, undocumented migrant field workers, or those trapped on cruise ships unable to dock? What about people with Down syndrome, schizophrenia, or, in general, people with disabilities of any kind?

Third, focus groups with impoverished Black and Latinx participants revealed that 83 percent would resist taking vaccines first or early.[29] Researchers at UAB spoke with 67 low-income people in eight focus groups in three Alabama counties and were surprised at the deep skepticism about taking Covid vaccines. The Kaiser Family Foundation discovered the same fact: one in three Black people would hesitate to take Covid vaccines, a fact that held steady for months into 2021.[30]

When Melinda Gates said that Black people deserved priority in getting vaccines because they were dying at twice the rate of whites, she had an unexpected reception in the Black community, when "many Black people viewed it as her advocating experimentation" on them.[31] In Ohio, 60 percent of the staff of nursing homes—which are overwhelmingly people of color—declined to be vaccinated, as did 30 percent in New York State.[32] In Britain, Black, Asian, and other minority groups resisted taking the vaccine.[33] In short, skepticism about Covid vaccines is pervasive and deep, and near-universal among people of color. This is the legacy of the Tuskegee syphilis study, of Henrietta Lacks, and of other racist incidents in medicine.[34] NIH Director Francis Collins said that the demonstrations in the summer of 2020 against the death of George Floyd "likely added to feelings of mistrust between minority groups and government or pharmaceutical companies,"[35] making it difficult for drug companies developing vaccines to recruit African Americans. Just as centuries of racial injustice cannot be easily undone, so distrust of people victimized by racism over centuries cannot be undone overnight. Similar skepticism has been found among the First Peoples, whose ancestors may have been given blankets infected with smallpox. The skepticism of Black, brown, and Native American people to vaccines partially explains why significant numbers of workers in health care refuse vaccines. They are often people of color, poorly paid aides in nursing homes, hospitals, and clinics, who believe that President Donald Trump did not have their welfare at heart when he rushed vaccines in Operation Warp Speed.

What about the 12 to 13 million undocumented immigrants working in the United States and Canada? Many of them work in food production close together and get infected at high rates. The Trump administration made undocumented immigrants fear deportation under the Public Charge rule, which threatened deportation for using public benefits. Some states wanted to track vaccination with driver's licenses, documents unavailable to such workers. One California Assemblyman warned that vaccination will only work under these conditions: "One, if farmworkers feel confident and safe in taking it, and two, if we're doing it across the board irrespective of immigration status."[36]

When executives at the largest US facilities running long-term-care homes required employees to take vaccines or lose their jobs, suspicion increased. Making vulnerable workers fear being fired is not the best way to overcome fear of vaccines.

DIFFERENCES IN EFFORTS TO CONTROL INFECTION IN DIFFERENT VULNERABLE GROUPS

Students living close together in dorms on campus resemble workers moving close together in an Amazon warehouse; K–12 children learning close together in some ways resemble those forced to live in detention centers for undocumented immigrants; college athletes playing together on a team in contact sports against other teams resemble prisoners and guards forced to live close together. Despite these similarities and despite the high degree of vulnerability to the coronavirus, societies have responded in different ways to testing, treating, and interacting with these different groups.

College students were much more likely to be tested, live apart, socially distance, and be supported in quarantine than many other "congregate populations," such as those in prisons, group homes for people with autism or cognitive disabilities, meat-packing plants, or stranded workers on cruise ships. College athletes were tested three times a week to control the virus and allow teams to continue to play, whereas many governors in states with meat-packing plants, and OSHA under the Trump administration, resisted any testing at all in such plants or any distancing. Women sorting apples in a packing warehouse in southern California did not get masks, distancing, or testing, even as SARS2 infected workers in neighboring farms.[37]

Children and Class Differences

Most children infected with SARS2 were not seriously ill, although infected children in K–12 systems could certainly infect their teachers and staff. By and large, any damage to children may have stemmed more from the lack of attending schools in person. Socially isolated teenagers were especially vulnerable. Las Vegas felt forced to resume in-person schooling after the 18th teenager in its county committed suicide, double the rate of the previous year.[38] Previously in decline, cigarette smoking increased in 2020, as did consumption of alcohol. Deaths from opioid overdoses, holding for years at 70,000 per calendar year in the United States, even before the pandemic hit had soared to 80,000 between March 2019 and March 2020. In Canada's British Columbia, during the summer of 2020 far more people died of opioid overdoses than Covid, prompting officials to declare a second public health emergency.[39]

Children in rich private schools generally kept attending in person because there was a better teacher-to-student ratio, smaller classes, and more resources. Children in public schools in big cities had to learn remotely, often with parents—or sometimes a single parent—struggling to pay rent. Teachers in Chicago resisted being forced to teach without vaccination, but then parents and columnists accused them of racism, ableism, and not caring about children.[40]

Athletes

The health of college athletes became a major ethical issue on some campuses, with critics questioning whether colleges had the best interests of student-athletes at heart. In universities with big-time football and basketball programs, revenues from television and tournaments paid many bills, and in smaller colleges in the NCAA's Division III that are not allowed to offer athletic scholarships, the promise of playing a sport became the main reason many athletes and their parents chose to pay tuition at those colleges.

In general, the more money that is involved, the greater the frequency and accuracy of the SARS2 testing. Professional basketball players living in a bubble in Orlando were still tested twice a day. Rules were enforced there to keep games reasonably free of infected players. For small colleges in Division II and III, requirements to test athletes three times a week sometimes were budget-breakers or simply impossible to meet, so the colleges canceled a whole season. Nevertheless, although numerous games had to be canceled, and some conferences didn't play at all, enough big-time football and basketball games occurred to ensure nominal college and professional seasons, at least for television. It is also true that some players exercised the NCAA option to opt out for a season without penalty. Whether such a move will really be without penalty on their teams remains to be seen. It is also true that most players did not want to sit out a season and wanted to take the risks of playing. The same was true of Olympic athletes hoping to compete in Japan in 2021.

As far as is known, no college athlete died after contracting Covid in contact sports. The long-term effects on infected athletes, especially regarding cardiac arrythmias, will eventually be understood. Especially troublesome is the existence of Long Covid among some athletes, where continuing fatigue is often the chief symptom and often derails an athlete's ability to perform.

FINAL NOTE

As we have seen, SARS2 thrives in those with weak immune systems who often have other health issues, as is the case for many of those in poverty. The impoverished often live in homeless shelters, which are further amplification systems. To lessen the impact of such amplification systems, we need to ensure that the homeless shelters have adequate PPE, handwashing stations, personnel, thermometers, and space. This may mean moving the most vulnerable to motels. If enough tests are available, residents should all be tested, and if this is not possible, they should be screened every day along with the staff. The poor have less access to care, often do not have primary care, and have less healthy habits, all of which make them an easier target for Covid.

Segregated housing, members of indigent families living in crowded conditions, and daily exposure to the virus without adequate PPE—these all contribute to the significant differences in infection from SARS2 and death from Covid among Latinx and Blacks. Communities must make certain that the less fortunate among them have access to health care, that they have SARS2 testing, and that, as vaccines become available, the most vulnerable are effectively encouraged to be vaccinated. In the midst of a pandemic, while reducing poverty should remain a fundamental goal, public-health workers should, at a minimum, educate the poor about Covid and explain the steps that they themselves can take to protect themselves.

The distribution of masks and hand sanitizers and the installation of portable sinks in areas where they are needed can reduce the impact of the pandemic. Where possible, alternative housing should be found for the homeless and for those in crowded homes, tents, or slums. Unemployment checks, food banks, and the CARES Act are also necessary to blunt the impact of the pandemic. Because these preventive and mitigation measures are complicated and expensive, government leadership and financing of these initiatives is required. We turn to the issue of pandemic leadership in the next chapter.

CHAPTER 12
LEADERSHIP DURING PANDEMICS

If it is the business of injustice to engender hatred wherever it is found, will it not, when it springs up either among free men or slaves, cause them to hate and be of strife with one another, and make them incapable of effective action in common?

—Socrates to Thrasymachus in *The Republic*[1]

Pandemics bring out the very best, and the very worst, of people.

—Laura Spinney, author of *Pale Rider*[2]

During the two centuries when ancient Rome was at the peak of its powers, it seemed destined to continue forever. Augustus, ruling from 27 BCE to 14 CE, created the Pax Romana (Roman Peace), which brought stability to the empire and culminated in the "Five Good Emperors" who ruled from 96–180 CE. Likewise, many citizens of developed countries take it for granted that, assuming good leadership, their countries will have a future. The history of leadership in the midst of pandemics suggests otherwise.

In the great Pulitzer Prize–winning social anthropologist Jared Diamond's book *Collapse: How Societies Choose to Fail or Succeed*,[3] he concentrates on societies that faced environmental threats and failed to meet them, such as that on the island of Hispaniola, shared by the countries of the Dominican Republic and Haiti. The former preserved its environment and created better leaders, whereas centuries of corrupt, crippling dictatorships destroyed Haiti's environment, economy, and social structures. In the absence of competent leadership, Haiti has always been on the verge of collapse.

This chapter discusses how good and bad leaders in 2020 confronted Covid. When faced with a major threat, good leaders rally citizens to fight. Bad leaders will not, or cannot, do the same, and pandemics may thus overwhelm their countries.

LEADERSHIP AND THE VIRTUE OF TRUST

A major kind of ethical theory not yet mentioned but important in fighting pandemics is virtue theory, which focuses not on universalizable rules (Kant), the best consequences (utilitarianism), or the good of those one cares about (care ethics), but on the character of a person. The theory dates back to Socrates, Plato, Aristotle, and other ancient Greek philosophers, who first systematically studied the *ethika aretai*, or excellent traits—what today we call "the virtues." These philosophers studied the virtues of courage (*andreia*) temperance (*sophrosyne*), justice (*dike*), and practical wisdom (*phronesis*). Later, Christianity added faith, hope, and charity to its list of cardinal virtues to create its classic Seven Virtues, as well as seven more theological virtues (chastity, humility, temperance, kindness, patience, diligence, charity). Later, for Kant and his upbringing in Christianity, the specific virtues became secondary to an overall character trait of simple virtue (from the Latin *virtus*), the inner desire to do the right action simply because one's rational self recognizes its inherent rightness. In this sense, one can distinguish between the virtues of the ancient Greeks and virtue in Kantian–Christian ethics.[4] Virtue theory studies both traits of character.

For the purposes of fighting pandemics, the virtue or virtues of leaders matters greatly. And when struggling with pandemics, one particular virtue stands out as important for good leaders: their trustworthiness. Pandemics require swift responses, sudden changes in normal behavior, and a need for cohesive group action. All of these actions require trust by the public that their politicians, scientists, and experts do not mislead them but guide them to safety. This virtue of trust is like health: you take it for granted until it's gone, and then you miss it terribly. It is almost impossible to exaggerate how many aspects of modern life assume trust. Take banking. Most people put their paychecks into banks and trust that their money will be there when they need it. When banks routinely failed or were robbed, as they were sometimes in the Wild West of America, citizens carried their money in gold or silver, making the risk of losing their money even greater.

Trust lies behind people putting away money for pensions for retirement, buying life insurance, buying long-term-care policies, and buying stocks and bonds. You trust institutions with your money, trusting that honorable people in them will do with it what they promised. In the United States, you allow money for social security to be deducted from your paycheck, trusting that later in your life, a pension from it will come to you. Trust also lies behind human communication. If most people routinely lied most of the time, nobody could believe anything easily and human actions would be curtailed. For example, if a sign at night says, "Bridge out ahead: take detour," and disbelieving drivers ignored the warning, disastrous consequences would obviously occur. When driving, you also trust that red lights work. Parents trust that teachers are screened, such that a monster does not teach their children. In colleges and universities, you trust that someone ensures the integrity of courses and degrees, that everything has not been watered down, that graduates are not going into debt for worthless degrees.

Trust matters in eating. If you eat a hamburger, you trust that the Department of Agriculture has not fired all its meat inspectors. You trust that rotten carcasses do not get made into hamburger. In restaurants, you trust that hamburgers are thoroughly cooked to prevent transmission of *E. coli*. With organic food, you trust that farmers, by themselves on a distant field away from prying eyes, don't use pesticides and chemical fertilizers to increase their yields. And trust matters in medicine. In the United States, where many specialists earn lucrative incomes based on the number of procedures they perform, you trust that your physician recommends a procedure not to augment his income but for your best interest. You trust drug companies not to lie about their data to the FDA.

During the AIDS crisis in the 1980s, Americans became angry when they realized that Joseph Bove, head of the American Red Cross, and Margaret Heckler, head of Health and Human Services, had lied to them about the blood supply being safe from HIV. Similarly, both supporters and opponents of Donald Trump became angry when they realized that he and his appointees had not been truthful with them about Covid. When the first American case occurred, he reassured Americans, "It's one person coming in from China. It's going to be fine."[5] Likewise, when CDC director Robert Redfield briefed 20 US Senators about outbreaks of the coronavirus, he reassured them, "We are prepared for this."[6]

Although Operation Warp Speed threw a lot of money at companies developing vaccines, the Trump administration did nothing to build the infrastructure to develop, distribute, monitor, regulate, and govern the distribution of vaccines, resulting in chaos in January 2021. Before the Biden administration began, no one was working to make sure vaccinations would work. Trust was betrayed.

THE WHO'S LEADERS MADE MISTAKES

Unfortunately, trusted leaders of the World Health Organization (WHO) made errors in confronting the Covid pandemic. First, they downplayed the seriousness of the virus, naïvely taking China's word as to its origins in a Wuhan market selling live animals and that no community spread had occurred. Critics say that the WHO was too indebted to China, which funded a good chunk of its budget, and was too afraid of alienating the Trump administration, which feared alarmism about the virus and which funded 20 percent of the WHO's budget. Second, the WHO failed to recognize and inform the public that masks not only reduced the spread of COVID for other people but also reduced both a person's own chance of contracting COVID and the severity of their case. If nothing else, the experience of Asian countries in previously fighting pandemics and where wearing masks in public had become a norm should have informed the WHO's views.

Third, the WHO's leaders initially claimed that transmission of Covid through asymptomatic individuals was rare. In mid-April 2020, several courageous physicians, including two young women in Germany, sounded the alarm that infected people could spread the virus two to three days before they showed symptoms.[7] Such "asymptomatic spread" was crucial to understanding how to slow the spread of the virus, because most initial efforts focused only on testing those with symptoms and on screening only for high temperatures. But if asymptomatic, infected individuals were spreading the virus two to three days before they had outward symptoms, new kinds of testing would be needed. After hundreds of scientists penned a letter about their beliefs in such transmission, the WHO finally relented. Eventually, people determined that 30 percent of transmission was asymptomatic. And fourth, the WHO initially emphasized that only droplets spread the virus. Compared to aerosols, droplets stay in the air for much less time and spread less than aerosols. As was later discovered, aerosols transmit the virus better than droplets, a fact the WHO only belatedly recognized.[8]

To its credit, the WHO established an independent panel to investigate these early responses to the pandemic, which agreed that the WHO had been too easy on China and had made mistakes, but also emphasized that the WHO lacked the funding, legal powers, and cooperation of leading nations to have prevented this outbreak and future ones. It also recommended limiting its director-general post to 7 years (to prevent campaigning) and establishing an international system to monitor and warn nations of outbreaks of infectious diseases.[9]

DONALD TRUMP AND AMERICAN LEADERSHIP

Donald Trump and Jacinda Ardern Confront a Pandemic

The presumed trustworthiness of a leader can be abused. Presumed trust makes it very easy for bad leaders to deceive citizens, as the following timeline comparing US president Donald Trump (in bold) and New Zealand prime minister Jacinda Ardern (in italics) makes clear.

Dec. 31, 2019   China announces 27 cases of a puzzling pneumonia in Wuhan; Taiwan tests all passengers arriving from Wuhan for a SARS-like virus and involuntarily quarantines anyone with symptoms.

Jan. 6, 2020   News that a mysterious pneumonia has appeared in Wuhan, China, tied to a wet-food market; it supposedly has killed no one and does not spread person to person.

Jan. 9   Science journalists Donald McNeil and Sui-Lee Wee break the story of a new coronavirus as cause of the outbreak.[10]

Jan. 13   First case outside China reported in Thailand, evidence of person-to-person spread.

Jan. 15   **First American case in Washington state: resident who returned from visit to Wuhan.**

Jan. 23   China extraordinarily quarantines 11 million citizens in Wuhan, indicating a dangerous virus.

Jan. 24   **Mark Pottinger, US Deputy National Security Advisor, warns President Trump of new virus.**

Jan. 25   CDC rejects German test for virus used by WHO; tries and fails to develop an accurate test.

Jan. 28   **Robert O'Brien, National Security Advisor, tells President that the new virus "will be the roughest thing you face" during his presidency.**

Jan. 31   **Trump bans incoming travel from China.**

Feb. 2   **Trump tells Sean Hannity of Fox News, "We have it [the virus] totally under control. It's one person coming in from China, and we have it under control. It's going to be just fine."**
New Zealand's Prime Minister, Jacinda Ardern, bans travel to/ from China.

Feb. 7   **Trump privately tells veteran journalist Bob Woodward about virus on tape that, "It goes through air. That's always tougher than the touch.... This is more deadly than the flu," in fact five times more so. "This is deadly stuff."[11]**

Feb. 27   **Trump publicly claims about virus, "One day—it's like a miracle—it will disappear."[12]**
First case in New Zealand: Ardern says her goal is to eliminate the virus from New Zealand.

March 1   WHO, CDC, and US Surgeon General Jerome Adams advise *against* wearing masks to prevent spread of the virus, telling citizens they only need to do so when near infected relatives.

March 8   Northern Italy overrun with cases; Prime Minister Conte locks down northern Italy for two months.

March 10   **States lack ventilators and PPE for doctors; Trump refuses to invoke Defense Production Act to produce more, telling states' governors, "Try getting it yourselves." Governors say they must flatter Trump to get PPE and ventilators from federal stockpiles.**[13]

March 19   California governor Gavin Newsom issues stay-at-home orders to 40 million, curtailing the virus's spread.
Ardern closes borders and imposes 14-day quarantine on all visitors.

March 25   *Ardern starts month-long Level 4 lockdown; says "We're all in this together." Requires mandatory mask wearing, distancing, mass testing.*

March 27   British prime minister Boris Johnson tests positive for SARS2 and is soon hospitalized.

April 3   **When asked about CDC's recommendation to wear cloth masks, President Trump replies: "It's voluntary. I don't think I'm going to be doing it." Makes not wearing masks symbolize supporting him.**

April 24   **Trump extols the virtues of bleach and ultraviolet light to cleanse away the virus and suggests investigations into internal uses of bleach through injection. Scientists mock the suggestion. President in turn mocks and undermines them.**[14]
Ardern works closely with scientists and public health officials.

April 28   **Trump publicly promises that testing in states will soon double; privately rants against testing.**[15]

May 27   **Editorial board of *USA Today*, with largest circulation of any American newspaper, says a "leadership failure" has caused 100,000 American deaths."**[16]

June 8   *Ardern reports that New Zealand has zero cases. The United States tops 2 million cases.*

June 10   Normal life resumes in Wuhan, with zero cases.

June 18   **As cases surge in 20 states, President Trump publicly claims that virus "is fading away."**[17]

July 17   Georgia governor Brian Kemp files lawsuit to prevent Atlanta's mayor from requiring masks.
New cases in the United States surpass 70,000 per day.

Aug. 11   *New Zealand, with population of 5 million, goes 100 days without one case of local transmission.*

Aug. 18   **Trump complains that testing for virus is "killing me! This whole thing is. We've got all the damn cases. I want to do what Mexico does. They don't give you a test until you go to the emergency room and you're vomiting."**[18]

Sept. 4 **Trump mocks Joe Biden for wearing a mask in public and the way he wears them.**
84 percent of New Zealanders approve of Ardern and are proud of New Zealand's success.

Sept. 7 **Trump asks a reporter asking question during press conference to remove his face mask: "If you don't take it off, you're very muffled."**

Sept. 26 **Super-spreader ceremony in Rose Garden for Judge Amy Coney Barrett infects many present.**

Sept. 28 One million deaths worldwide.

Oct. 3 **Trump tests positive for virus and enters hospital. Wife, youngest son, dozens of staff also positive.**

Oct. 7 **Trump leaves hospital and removes mask symbolically on White House balcony while talking to mask-less supporters below; compares himself to Superman for having beaten the virus.**

Oct. 14 **Veteran epidemiologist Larry Brilliant says Trump's "colossal failure of leadership" caused extra 150,000 Americans to die.[19]**
New Trump medical appointee Dr. Scott Atlas vehemently opposes expanded testing.[20]
Trump refuses to release $9 billion earmarked for expanded testing for virus.

Oct. 17 *Ardern easily wins second term as prime minister in national election.*

Nov. 9 **Trump loses presidential election to Joe Biden. His handling of pandemic is a big issue.**

Nov. 10 Second Covid wave in Europe forces countries into lockdown again.

Dec. 14 **First American vaccinated; Trump HHS secretary promises 20 million vaccinations by end of month; only 2 million get vaccinated.**
China claims it defeated virus; says **Trump's failure with virus made the United States a "defeated power."[21]**
Life normalizes for most Chinese citizens as 2021 begins; China reports only 100,000 cases.[22]

Jan. 19, 2021 **Trump's last day as President; he leaves Biden with 24,000,000 cases, 400,000 deaths, and a deeply divided country.**

May 15 **US has 32,900,000 cases, 585,000 deaths.**
New Zealand has 2,645 cases, 26 deaths.

185

Trump Undermines the CDC, Pressures the FDA, Withdraws from WHO

As the virus rampaged in Italy in March 2020, early in the pandemic, a press conference occurred where Nancy Messonnier, Director of the National Center for Immunization and Respiratory Diseases at the CDC, reported that she had asked the principal of her children's school what plans had been made for remote teaching because the coronavirus would soon shut down in-person classes. The next day, the stock market fell steeply, and Nancy Messonnier was not heard from again in public for the rest of 2020. After Biden became president, the truth emerged: Trump had banned Messonnier from speaking again.[23]

Early in his presidency, Donald Trump had appointed Robert Redfield to lead the CDC, an unpopular choice within the agency and an elderly, reclusive man who preferred to lead from his home outside Washington, DC, rather than his official office at the CDC in Atlanta. Through much of the pandemic, Redfield seemed content to let Trump appointees change or massage CDC's recommendations and bulletins. In trying to create its own Covid test, the CDC had made a terrible mistake by not accepting the German test used by the WHO and the rest of the globe. This mistake resembled the mistake in the 1980s when France wanted its own test for HIV and delayed testing its hemophiliacs; as a result, for six months France was unable to test its hemophiliac population for HIV infection from medically necessary blood transfusions. Similarly, it took a precious month for the CDC to iron out problems in its own Covid test, a month that allowed the coronavirus to seed itself all over the United States. While in early March 2020, South Korea was testing 10,000 people a day to defeat the virus, the United States in April struggled to test 10,000 a week.

After American passengers on the Diamond Princess had been released from quarantine, Trump officials chartered two planes to fly Americans home. They were quarantined upon arriving at Travis Air Force Base in northern California. Although career scientists at the CDC vigorously protested, infected Americans were flown on the same plane as Americans free of the virus, and all shared the same toilet and air. Later, several Americans who boarded the plane negative became infected, as CDC staffers had predicted would happen. The Trump administration also dispatched a dozen workers from Health and Human Services to greet the passengers upon their arrival (which critics saw as the president wanting to take credit for their rescue).[24] Unfortunately, these HHS workers did not wear PPE and they then patronized motels and restaurants around the base. A week or so later, cases predictably erupted around that base.

In an ominous development in mid-July, the Trump administration gutted the CDC and announced that, henceforth, its own staff in Washington, DC, would collect and announce data about COVID infections and deaths.[25] When the CDC's evisceration was announced, the United States had 4 million known infections and 140,000 deaths. Yet because it was so hard to get a test, no one knew the true number of infected Americans, although some estimates projected that as many as 40 million Americans had already been infected.[26] Also during that summer, a CDC plan for safely re-opening schools was gutted from 23 pages of details to six pages of vague exhortations. Despite growing evidence from South Korea that children, although they rarely got sick, could easily spread the virus to their parents and grandparents,[27] the Trump administration pressed all schools in all states to re-open normally, thus creating potential amplification systems in every community. While many teachers worried about getting infected while teaching or infecting their families, some parents publicly protested to have all schools re-open.

Before the Covid pandemic began, Trump had already fired or restricted career scientists at the Food and Drug Administration (FDA) and the Environmental Protection Agency (EPA), as well as at the CDC, replacing the heads of these institutions with men who would institute his dismissive policies about Covid testing and reporting. Each of these new health chiefs made the problems of testing Americans worse: Stephen Hahn, the head of the FDA, denied universities and private labs the right to make better tests; Alex Azar, head of the Health and Human Services Administration (HHS) refused (with Trump) to invoke the Defense Production Act (DPA) to compel American manufacturers to make scarce ventilators and other supplies. Even six months after the first case in the United States, the Trump administration had still not invoked the DPA to make much-needed swabs, testing reagents, and personal protective equipment (PPE). When Trump fired scientists who failed to do his bidding and replaced them with those who would at the FDA and the CDC, as head of HHS, and as Surgeon General, physicians and citizens began to distrust the new officials. Robert Redfield allowed bulletins about the coronavirus to be censored and rewritten by members of Trump's staff, while Surgeon General Jerome Adams dismissed concerns about Covid, saying it was only a flu.[28]

When Anthony Fauci said publicly, "Re-opening too soon can create something you can't control," Trump attacked him. Anyone who disagreed with him publicly, such as Dr. Rick Bright, four-year director of BARDA (the Biomedical Advanced Research and Development Authority), who warned that the country was not controlling the virus and that deaths would be catastrophic, was punished. In Bright's case, he was re-assigned to meaningless work that left him idle for weeks until he finally resigned. Like Trump, Republican governors in Arizona, Georgia, Florida, Iowa, Nebraska, and Alabama seemed to suppress the number of infections and deaths, or at least made no real efforts to get accurate numbers. That fueled major spread of the virus because if you don't know where it's exploding, you can't mount efforts to contain it.

Leadership Battles over PPE and Ventilators

The United States was ill prepared for this pandemic, despite years of warnings by experts that one was inevitable. Supplies of PPE were quickly exhausted. In contrast, and before it realized the scale of the pandemic, Germany was too confident, actually exporting millions of masks and PPE clothing to other countries. In the United States, instead of unity through a national plan to defeat Covid, Trump made governors compete against each other for supplies and for favors. Thus, states were on their own, bidding against one another for PPE made in China. In one instance, Massachusetts ordered 3 million masks, only to see them seized in New York Harbor by the federal government for its own dwindling cache. So crazy did leadership battles become among state governors that when a plane landed at Baltimore's airport with a half million COVID tests from South Korea, the Republican governor of Maryland, Larry Hogan, had to make Maryland State Police and the National Guard meet the plane and hide the tests in a secret location, lest federal agents swoop in and take them.[29]

Why? Although the Trump administration couldn't get its act together to actually order such tests, or create them, it wasn't above stealing them from states that bought them elsewhere. In Florida, federal agents seized masks intended for firefighters in Miami-Dade County. When the federal government did dispatch PPE from its stockpile, the PPE was sometimes rotten, as was true of 500 masks delivered to Montgomery County, Alabama. Such was the disarray of the American response to obtain supplies to fight the pandemic.[30]

On April 2, 2020, Trump finally invoked the DPA to force companies to make ventilators (and only to make ventilators). And PPE? Well, again, like testing and distribution of vaccines later, that was up to the states to obtain.

Scapegoating

Names of epidemics and the agents that cause them are frequently ideological. Recall that the early name for HIV/AIDS was "Gay Related Immune Deficiency," or GRID. As historians Alan Brandt and Alyssa Botelho observe, even to call the Covid pandemic "a perfect storm" had political implications because it implied that the new virus could have been neither predicted nor better prepared for.[31] To the contrary, numerous books, commissions, and studies had long predicted a viral pandemic such as SARS2.[32]

President Trump blamed everybody for the virus but himself: he blamed the Chinese, calling the virus "the Kung Flu" and "the Chinese virus."[33] His followers sometimes called it "the Wuhan virus," such as Texas Congressman Louie Gohmert, who often did not wear a mask and who championed not doing so, got COVID and, bizarrely, blamed his rare use of his cloth mask for infecting him.[34] Some people believe that these comments led to a wave of new violence against Asians in the United States, nearly 4,000 incidents.[35]

Finally, in the digital age, the media has become a gargantuan amplification system. A century ago, during the Spanish flu pandemic in 1918, newspapers accepted ads for quack treatments for influenza. Sadly, today it is far more than just newspapers that spread faulty information. Partisan news outlets such as Fox News and citizens on social media (including the president himself) spread misinformation and disinformation. Trump also blamed the WHO and halted American money to fund it. He blamed the "liberal media" for exaggerating the numbers and severity of Covid. He blamed Democratic leaders, such as Nancy Pelosi and Andrew Cuomo, for undermining him, when in reality he constantly undermined them.

Two Similar States with Two Different Leaders: Vermont and South Dakota

South Dakota has 884,000 citizens; Vermont has 624,000. South Dakota is 86-percent white, Vermont, 94-percent. Both have Republican governors, college towns, and many rural residents, but South Dakota has nearly 10 times more infections and deaths than Vermont. Why? Because two leaders—two governors—led in different ways during the pandemic.

South Dakota governor Kristi Noem opposed lockdowns, face masks, and stay-at-home orders, claiming they didn't work and violated residents' freedoms. An outbreak at a meat-packing plant in Sioux Falls in April 2020 created 3,000 cases, and the subsequent motorcycle rally in Sturgis that summer created more. By February 2021, South Dakota had the second-highest infection rate in the United States per capita by state.

In contrast, Vermont's governor Phil Scott, like New Zealand's prime minister Jacinda Ardern, aggressively fought the virus, aiming to totally eliminate it. In March, he closed schools and businesses, issued stay-at-home orders, ordered mask wearing in public, and made visitors quarantine for 14 days before interacting with Vermonters. He declared a state of emergency from mid-March to mid-September, giving state police and National Guard troops guidelines for enforcement of Vermont's rules.

Date	VERMONT Cases	Deaths	SOUTH DAKOTA Cases	Deaths
March 7, 2020	1	0	0	0
March 11	1	0	8	0
March 31	293	13	108	1
July 16	1,334	56	7,694	115
October 4	1,785	58	24,418	248
December 9	5,285	86	88,023	1,147
December 28	7,120	87	98,158	1,446
January 18, 2021	10,321	163	105,659	1,677
May 14	23,792	252	123,644	1,991

JUDGMENT OF US LEADERS DURING THE PANDEMIC

Various research organizations surveyed people around the world about how world leaders handled the Covid pandemic. The Pew Research Center surveyed people in 13 nations and discovered in September 2020 that views of American leaders had dropped to historic lows, with unfavorable views by 59 percent of those in Britain, 69 percent of those in France, 74 percent of Germans, 65 percent of Canadians, and 67 percent of Australians.[36] Reuters News Service found that 60 percent of the world's people agreed that China had responded well to the pandemic, but only a third thought that the United States had.[37] People in Greece, Taiwan, Ireland, South Korea, Australia, and Denmark thought their leaders had handled the crisis well. By September, only 15 percent of people around the world agreed that the United States had done a good job handling the virus.

Although it irritated many Americans to hear it, the mishandling of the pandemic by the United States dismayed people around the world: "I feel sorry for Americans," said a member of Myanmar's parliament, a sentiment echoed by the mayor of Sarnia, a Canadian city on the border with Michigan: "Personally, it's like watching the decline of the Roman Empire."[38] While 99 percent of China's citizens in 2021 could attend concerts, conferences, and gatherings of up to a thousand people, citizens of North America increasingly experienced lockdowns and feared infection from each other. A Western businessman visiting Beijing and Shanghai in 2021 ironically observed that it "felt a bit like the Epcot Center at Disney...like a microcosm of the West is still here, but the West is shut down at the moment."[39]

In terms of trust in world leaders, Angela Merkel was most trusted, followed by Emmanuel Macron in France. Not trusted were Vladimir Putin of Russia and Xi Jinping of China, followed by the least-trusted leader, Donald Trump.[40] Women everywhere trusted Donald Trump much less than men did.

FINAL NOTE

What can be learned from comparing the failure of the United States to contain the virus with the success of other countries such as New Zealand? As the *New England Journal of Medicine* summarized,

> Rapid, science-based risk assessment linked to early, decisive government action was critical. Implementing interventions at various levels (border-control measures, community-transmission control measures, and case-based control measures) was effective. Prime Minister Jacinda Ardern [in New Zealand] provided empathic leadership and effectively communicated key messages to the public—framing combating the pandemic as the work of a unified "team of 5 million"—which resulted in

high public confidence and adherence to a suite of relatively burdensome pandemic-control measures.[41]

As the United States hit a half-million Covid deaths on February 22, 2021, Anthony Fauci observed that one hundred years from now, the Trump administration's failure to control the coronavirus will go down in history as the greatest failure in public health of modern times: "If you look back historically [over 2020], we've done worse than almost any other country," he said.[42] Many countries around the world with leaders who unified their countries did so much better: Senegal, Vietnam, and Rwanda. Bhutan, a country of 700,000 with an open border with India, has had one Covid death.

If there is leadership and lack of leadership, Mr. Trump's failures with the pandemic go beyond lack of leadership to something darker, perhaps something we should call "anti-leadership." Almost everything he did, from delaying production of PPE, to delaying testing, to weaponizing supplies, to politicizing vaccine production, to promoting large, unmasked crowds, helped the virus spread. Even when he and his family became infected, even with half the staff in the White House infected, he refused to lead.

CHAPTER 13
THE FUTURE

This book was finished in early 2021, but long-term outcomes of COVID-19 are uncertain, so much of the following summarizes various speculations about what might occur in 2021–22 and beyond.

THE FUTURE OF COVID-19

Michael Osterholm and his colleagues at Minnesota's Center for Infectious Disease Research and Policy describe three possible scenarios for SARS2.[1] The first follows the course of the Spanish flu of 1918: a small wave in the spring of 2020, followed by a huge, lethal wave eight to nine months later of more infectious, lethal variants, then two years of tapering during which a less lethal variant evolves that is only like a bad flu. In this scenario, changes in the virus itself and its hosts make the virus weaken in virulence, as happened with swine flu in 1976 and with MERS. A second scenario predicts a rollercoaster of peaks and valleys over the same period, but at the end, the coronavirus also weakens. The final scenario is slow burn, during which, after an initial period of intense infection, small peaks and valleys of outbreaks occur around the world indefinitely.[2] In other words, the virus and its variants would become endemic in the United States and other countries around the world, nestled in pools of infection that might create new variants.

As several such new variants emerged in 2021, former CDC director Tom Frieden endorsed the third scenario, saying the world needed to go through the five stages of grief, get past denial, anger, depression, and bargaining, and move to accepting the fact that SARS2 viruses will be with us for years, if not decades, becoming endemic like HPV, HIV, Zika, rabies, and malaria—in short, moving from being a pandemic to being endemic, varying in intensity in different countries across the globe, permanently altering our way of life.[3] Boris Johnson warned the British public in late February 2021, "There is ... no credible route to a zero-Covid Britain or indeed a zero-Covid world,"[4] meaning everyone should expect periodic outbreaks, new variants, continued masking, and yearly vaccinations. In a webinar the same month, Anthony Fauci agreed that the virus will likely become endemic and not disappear soon.

All three scenarios predict at least two more years for the toll of the coronavirus and its variants on humans. The slow-burn scenario involves even more years. If any of these are correct, then the Covid pandemic will change us in many ways. It is also possible that by the end of 2021, the world will create many effective vaccines, including affordable ones, possibly even ones that give sterilizing immunity, and SARS2 and its variants will be stopped.

Vaccines against SARS2 Every Year?

Testing, tracing, and isolation failed in the West partly because, as Fareed Zakaria said, "People in the West can't be disciplined enough to isolate themselves and prevent infection of others." For this reason, says Devi Sridhar, Professor of Public Health and Chair of Global Medicine at the University of Edinburgh, "the West, where the virus is endemic, will need to roll out new vaccines or booster vaccines every year to create some kind of normal."[5] Pfizer's CEO confirmed this view on April 15, 2021, when he predicted that people getting his vaccine would need a booster 12 months after their second shot and probably an annual booster every year after that.[6] That prediction fueled more worries about vaccine nationalism because officials worried that plants manufacturing vaccines would be tied up making boosters for citizens of developed countries while ignoring the developing world. But allowing much of the world to go unvaccinated would also allow variants to flourish. Professor Sridhar worried especially about the South African variant, which seemed to reinfect people previously infected with the original SARS2 virus from Wuhan. Moreover, as London epidemiologist Deepti Gurdasani emphasized in 2020, "There are problems not just with the procurement of vaccines. We don't know how long their efficacy will last.... This idea that Covid will end by summer or by the end of next year, it's frankly ridiculous."[7]

In the slow-burn scenario, large reservoirs of SARS2 and its variants will exist in conjunction with large reservoirs of uninfected people. Such conditions will allow variants of SARS2 to emerge. The B117 ("U.K.") variant jumped in one month from 20 percent of the cases in Britain to 90 percent. Cases of the same variant in the United States by May 8, 2021, comprised 72% of the thousands of new daily cases, 70% in Michigan, and were expected to soon dominate, along with other new variants specific to New York and Oregon.[8] Pfizer started a study in February to see if a third dose would protect against variants, and Moderna started a trial of a new vaccine against the South African strain. New vaccines against SARS2 may be quadrivalent, protecting against four strains, like current flu vaccines. Current vaccines protect only against Covid and do not offer sterilizing immunity against acquiring SARS2. We don't know, in fact, whether sterilizing immunity is necessary: Salk's polio vaccine didn't provide such immunity, but it still helped stamp out polio in North America.

It is also worth recalling what it means to say that the Pfizer or Moderna vaccine is "95 percent" or "96 percent effective" against hospitalization and death, which is that some small percentage of those vaccinated will still be hospitalized or die. On April 13, 2021, the CDC reported that 5,814 Americans had been infected with SARS2 after vaccination, and of them, 396 were so sick that they required hospitalization and died.[9] If nothing else, this statistic shows that even the best vaccinations are not "Get Out of Jail Free" cards to cease taking precautions against infection.

One obstacle to herd immunity is children, who in the United States constitute 25 percent of the population and who can still transmit virus. Pfizer is testing a vaccine on children aged 12–16, but others will be needed for younger children. Mandatory vaccination may be required in the United States to reach herd immunity, but until vaccines get approval for regular, non-emergency use, such a requirement will face legal challenges.[10] A waitress in New York City, for example, who was fired for refusing to vaccinate, promptly consulted an employment and labor lawyer.[11]

* * * * *

Note: For the remainder of this discussion of the future, let's assume that SARS2 does not miraculously disappear in 2021, that large parts of the globe contain reservoirs of vulnerable, uninfected people, and that new variants occasionally emerge. These assumptions underlie the discussions that follow.

For Long Covid, How Long?

A significant impact of the coronavirus pandemic will be the number of long-haulers and how their lives go. If billions on the planet become infected, and if a quarter of them still experience symptoms six months later, the damage of SARS2 will extend far beyond the lives lost, with severe economic, medical, and social consequences for the millions with long-term impairments who lack the security of a national health system.

Major medical centers already offer special clinics for Covid long-haulers. The NIH and WHO should fund long-term studies of such patients. One special problem is whether long-haulers have immunity to new infections from variants. Long-haulers also create special problems for vaccination certificates. If long-haulers continue to host SARS2, even in a reservoir organ, should their freedoms be restricted? Studies should be done to see if they can pass the virus to others, especially through intimate contact. If enough people emerge with Long Covid, their status and issues may be one of the most significant ethical issue to emerge from the Covid pandemic.

Different Countries Will Deal with Outbreaks in Different Ways

Devi Sridhar, cited above, also says, "It is useful to think of Covid not as a single global pandemic, but as a simultaneous outbreak of innumerable local epidemics, each one slightly different."[12] She also predicts that "different countries will approach the future in different ways. New Zealand will try to eliminate the virus inside its borders."[13] Indeed, Asian countries will likely do better in controlling the virus than those in the West, especially Western countries with porous borders. Authoritarian governments will likely contain the virus better than ones emphasizing individual liberties. If people won't isolate, testing and contact tracing become pointless. But some democracies use muscle to triumph over the virus: in South Korea, if you break quarantine, you go to jail or get fined a large amount.

If pandemics cause enough economic damage, China and the East may rise economically while Europe and North America may suffer. Future economic prosperity may involve not investing in guns or bombs but successfully fighting pandemics. Some rich nations may become lone wolves, turning inward and ignoring the less fortunate of the world. Racism and tribalism may foster such moves; even strong national identities that are helpful because they foster a sense that "we're all in this together" may become counterproductive by fostering the national sentiment that "it's us against the world." Japan banned foreign tourists from its 2021 summer Olympics, hoping to control the virus. Under the guise of keeping Covid out, countries may focus more and more on keeping their country safe.

Gaps between Rich and Poor May Increase

According to the World Bank, the last eight months of 2020 erased four years of economic prosperity in the world, and for the first time in 20 years, the world's economies shrank.[14] As a result, at least 90 million people were thrown into extreme poverty, a number sure to double or triple by the end of 2021. Global warming has already destroyed the ability of many people in Central and South America to make a living as farmers. Crime in such places and the uncontrolled virus will likely push millions north, seeking escape and a better life in the United States and Canada. Paradoxically, because many of the world's poor are young and undernourished, they will not die from Covid, but pandemics will intensify their food insecurity, especially in developing countries in Africa, South America, and parts of Asia, perhaps leading to the exodus of millions for safer countries.

Bill and Melinda Gates argue that rich countries cannot ignore poor countries, whose economies have been severely damaged from declines in tourism. Nevertheless, Britain's success with the vaccines and the lack of it in the European Union vindicated those favoring Brexit, saying it allowed Britain to chart its own path, following Israel and the United States as vaccine leaders. Countries with strong national systems for public health and medical care will fare best. Otto von Bismarck correctly foresaw that a country is only as strong as the health of its population. In a pandemic, if wealthy owners of factories escape to safe island hideaways, leaving a mass of sick and vulnerable workers, the economy will suffer.

GAVI, the WHO, and developing countries pinned their hopes on the Astra-Zeneca vaccine, but this vaccine continued to have many problems, including confusing data presented to the US FDA, an inability to fulfill orders to Europe, a scare about blood clots that led to a pause in Europe and skepticism about it there, and a poor showing in South Africa against its variant. These problems bode poorly for a world hoping for this cheap vaccine.

Inside countries, similar gaps between rich and poor may widen. Tech savvy, well-off people may find ways to vaccinate themselves and their adult children, while poor, rural folks go without, creating a vaccinated elite who can travel freely and a mass of poor, vulnerable people who cannot. If highly aggressive or highly contagious variants make new vaccines necessary every year, will this gap widen even further? If a new quadrivalent vaccine against four strains of SARS2 becomes necessary, how long will it take to vaccinate most of the world? Over time, will environmental gaps become wider, hardened in the biology of vaccinations?

Higher Education May Change
College education may never be the same. In recent years, New York University has rebranded itself as a global university in which its undergraduates could spend a year in one of its 16 global campuses, from Shanghai to London, from Buenos Aires to Abu Dhabi. In 2020, that in-place global learning became mainly virtual for NYU students, but at least they studied with students from all over the world. In 2022, that trend will accelerate in online programs.

The online master's degree in Global Health at UAB already has graduate students from Washington, DC, California, and Nigeria, a trend that will grow among many MBA programs. It is also likely that leaders in high-quality online education such as Arizona State University will experience phenomenal growth because some professors and students discovered they prefer online classes. Pressure will increase to make online teaching not a profitable throw-away for students and faculty but an intensive, high-value experience. Some colleges will re-invent the Oxford tutorial, where a professor meets a student once a week to assign reading and go over essays written on the previous week's reading. Faculty who are teaching from home may resist being forced back on campus, especially if reservoirs of infection exist.

If the virus stays around in isolated clusters, periodically flaring up and infecting locals, parents and high-school students may disvalue out-of-state colleges, opting instead for a school that is close to home. But if classes stay only online, and students don't get awesome libraries, science labs, climbing walls, faculty-led travel abroad, clubs on campuses, opportunities on campus to join in research, and athletic teams, what are families paying $60,000 a year for? Some small, private colleges, dependent on such students to pay tuition and to live on campus, will need to change to survive. Going to college from home and hybrid classes on campuses are likely here to stay. If the virus lingers, home schooling will increase. Families may form pods, hiring good teachers and socializing only inside their pod.

If the virus stays around, academic conferences may incorporate Zoom audiences, even when in-person. People with physical disabilities and people without travel budgets can easily attend conferences online in ways they cannot with face-to-face meetings. Although many important things are lost by not meeting face-to-face, other things are gained, such as being able to anonymously zip from one session to another to see what's going on, something that's awkward to do in person. No, that is not for everybody, but graduate students looking for jobs, who previously felt uncomfortable socializing with hiring faculty in smokey bars over drinks might feel more comfortable socializing in a Zoom breakout room. Monthly faculty committees with 20 members can more easily find a common time to meet on Zoom than in-person on campus. It can be easier for students and professors to have a ten-minute check-up meeting on Zoom than in an office.

Social Changes

Pulitzer Prize–winning science writer Laurie Garrett predicts that, just as the United States did not return to normal plane travel after the bombing of the World Trade Center, so the pandemic will change some practices forever. People will "re-evaluate the importance of travel. They'll revisit their use of mass transit. They'll revisit the need for face-to-face meetings."[15] In the first twelve months of the pandemic, 44 percent of Americans worked remotely and many wanted to continue, which some companies like Google, Slack, and Microsoft allowed, thereby saving on relocation expenses, costs of office space, while seeing productivity increase. With interest rates at historic lows, 26 million Americans planned to buy their first home in 2021, fueling mass migration from big cities with crowd diseases to safer suburbs and rural towns and creating perhaps the most significant change wrought by the pandemic.

If vaccines don't give sterilizing immunity, and variants persist, public life in North America and Europe in 2022 may soon look like life in the East, where everyone wears a mask, where people shun those coughing or showing signs of illness, and where people will pay extra for physically distanced travel, gyms, concerts, and education. Contactless credit cards are here to stay, as are self-service kiosks at grocery stores and pharmacies where customers may scan items and pay with no human interactions.

If variants of the virus persist, dating and casual affairs will need to take into account not only the possibility of sexually transmitted diseases such as HIV but also the likelihood of SARS2 infections. Dating apps such as OK Cupid and Tinder already report that users who disclose they've been vaccinated get liked at twice the rate of users who say they won't get any vaccine.[16] Immunity certificates will create new communities on dating apps, and laws may be passed criminalizing the use of fraudulent immunity certificates. On campuses with large numbers of fraternities and sororities, parties will struggle not to be super-spreader events.

LESSONS TO LEARN

The Limits of Professionalism

The work of medical staff during the Covid pandemic has been presented by the media through the lens of heroism and wartime metaphors: a troop of weary, brave medical staff fighting with few weapons against a fierce enemy. Although somewhat accurate, this lens has diverted attention from the ethical issue of the limits of compassionate professionalism in caring for Covid patients needing long, intensive care. As ICUs filled up and as staff became infected, tired, and overwhelmed, such intensive care for so long for so many patients could not continue indefinitely. One year into the pandemic, more and more staff quit or became infected, with 20 percent of US nursing homes reporting severe shortages. Also, because they were exposed to high levels of SARS2, long-haulers in medical professions suffered more than other long-haulers, and for longer durations.[17]

Quietly, of course, triage occurred, if nothing other than through the exhaustion of the staff in overwhelmed hospitals. With Covid patients aged 80 to 100 suffering multiple medical problems, ethical lines needed to be drawn about whether staff should do everything possible to keep such patients alive. At some point, medical futility enters, and the likelihood of a return to normal life becomes vanishingly small. At this point, staff need two things: clear ethical guidelines for cessation of treatment to relieve guilt in doing so, and legal immunity for doing so. This is crucial in states that require CPR in the absence of a signed DNR order.

Covid-deniers and anti-vaxxers also test the limits of professionals, especially when such patients not only refuse to admit they were mistaken but also refuse to admit in the hospital that they actually have Covid. If a patient refuses oxygen or a ventilator because "I don't have Covid," can staff overrule them for their own good? Does such a claim make a Covid-denier ipso facto incompetent? As the pandemic wears on, absence of clean, good PPE continues to be a major issue in many medical units, especially rural ones. Without good, appropriate PPE, staff cannot be required to do everything possible for every Covid patient. As many as four thousand American medical staff have become infected caring for Covid patients—how many of them became infected because of lack of good PPE?

As a field, bioethics began in 1962 by exposing ethical issues formerly discussed only privately inside medicine. In 2021, bioethics needs to serve the public and medicine again by creating national discussions of the limits of care of Covid patients in a world of scarce resources. The first year of the Covid pandemic moved issues dangerously the wrong way, from public discussion of allocation of ICU beds to private discussions inside hospitals.

Broken Agencies Need to Be Rebuilt

In 2021, the Independent Panel for Pandemic Preparedness and Research, an international organization, faulted the World Health Organization for not being prepared to stop the coronavirus that broke out in Wuhan in late 2019.[18] Besides suffering from a weak international bureaucracy and reporting laws in many countries that lacked teeth, the major problem was a philosophical paradox: the very brakes that had been put on the WHO to prevent alarmist warnings about spreading germs and that were feared to unnecessarily hurt the world's economies also prevented the WHO from acting more swiftly about the new coronavirus. Although the WHO had spent hundreds of millions of dollars to build an alarm system against coming pandemics, its bureaucracy and rules prevented it from being effective against SARS2.[19] As new viruses and their variants appear, the world will need to decide what it fears most: new pandemics or new crashes of the global economy.[20]

In early 2021, the Biden administration appointed Rochelle Walensky as the new director of the Centers for Disease Control, and she vowed to restore trust in the CDC.[21] Walensky headed the Department of Infectious Diseases at Massachusetts General Hospital, run by Harvard Medical School doctors, and enjoyed immense respect from fellow physicians and researchers around the world. The Biden administration also directed Anthony Fauci to lead the US effort to rejoin both the World Health Organization and Predict, a worldwide program with the new name of Spillover, whose goal was to predict outbreaks of new viruses from bat caves, wet markets, and wildlife-smuggling places.[22] Still, much work needs to be done to prepare for future pandemics.[23]

The backbone of public health in the United States is 3,000 state and local public-health departments, but these have been underfunded for decades, and in 2018 they had at least 38,000 and maybe as many as 56,000 fewer workers than in 2008.[24] The American system was so fragmented that the Dean of Columbia University's School of Public Health has argued that it will need a twenty-first-century Marshall Plan to rebuild it.[25] A survey by Kaiser Health News (KHN) and the Associated Press (AP) found that many hard-hit cities had cut staff at public-health departments. In 2009, Detroit had 700 employees, but in 2020 it had only 200. Outside big cities and rich coastal states, more than a fifth of public-health workers, the backbone of the "system" in the heartland of the United States from Ohio to Arizona, from Idaho to Mississippi, on average earned less than $35,000 a year.

Because of the attack on expertise under the Trump administration, public-health officials who tried to do their jobs and implement the standard rules against viral spread came under intense attack in many conservative states. In the spring of 2020, 38 leaders in such counties and states quit or were fired, the KHN/AP review found. So extreme was the vitriol against public health in the United States that in some states such as Idaho, politicians and public-health officials who voted to require residents to wear masks received death threats to themselves and their children. (Anthony Fauci had white powder mailed to his home, not knowing if it was anthrax or ricin, or if it was harmless.)

Current American culture is not equipped to fight new pandemics. Trust and support for public health may take decades to rebuild, and this rebuilding must entail the capacity to create accurate tests quickly for new viruses, the ability to do sentinel testing and to do genomic sequencing of viruses the way the United Kingdom does, the ability to identify who flew on airplanes and might be exposed to a new virus, and the ability to quarantine in hotels, at government expense, those exposed for 14 days, the way numerous countries do.

And the United States needs more than just more investment in public-health programs. Every other developed country of the world has a national medical system. Israel used its system, for example, to quickly vaccinate its citizens. Pandemics prove the urgent need for such national systems, but they cannot be created overnight. A national medical system such as Canada's has a record for each patient that is usually electronic, and such systems make it much easier to quickly identify who needs vaccination first and who has been vaccinated. As New York Times columnist Nicholas Kristoff concluded, "The United States is in a weaker position than some other countries to confront the virus because it is the only advanced country that doesn't have universal health coverage, and the only one that does not guarantee paid sick leave. With chronic diseases, the burden of these gaps is felt primarily by the poor; with infectious diseases, the burden will be shared by all Americans."[26]

Addressing Inequalities

Vaccine hesitancy can be overcome in people of color in various ways. Special vaccination vans in under-served neighborhoods and rural towns have proved useful, making it easy to get vaccines for ambivalent citizens. Famous athletes, actors, and local leaders can be vaccinated on television or in front of safe gatherings, leading the way. While specifically prioritizing people for vaccines or treatment by race may be unjustified, a better strategy seems to be that of Long Beach, California, which included exposed workers in nursing homes, grocery stores, buses, and schools in early groups for vaccination. Beyond 2021, perhaps the pandemic will finally move the United States to create a national system of medical care. Countries with such systems not only did better fighting the pandemic; they also did better in not letting the pandemic worsen inequalities. Such a national system needs public-health departments in each county, linked in a coherent national system.

Planning for future pandemics must include planning for childcare. Lack of affordable child care will hit families of color hard. If variants infect children, child-care centers may become unsustainable at reasonable costs, intensifying the need for one parent to stay at home when many couldn't afford to do so. If variants create the need for more lockdowns of schools, children of color will fall behind even more.

Jump on New Outbreaks Fast; Vaccinate Fast

The Biogen Conference in Boston shows what happens with a lackadaisical approach to outbreaks. Studies that traced SARS2 from that conference show that its attendees infected over 300,000 Americans.[27] Countries in the East, such as China, Hong Kong, Taiwan, and Australia, with their long experience with pandemics, stomp down hard on outbreaks, closing cities, borders, and airports and doing everything possible to contain the new germ. In 2021, new outbreaks in areas around Beijing led China to quarantine 22 million people there and discourage Chinese citizens from traveling soon after for the Lunar New Year.[28]

Despite the many faults of the Trump administration throughout the pandemic, it did one thing right: it procured a lot of vaccines for Americans, and even though it had no plan to get them into Americans' arms, the process was superior to the bureaucracy and in-fighting of the European Union that undercut the successes of Germany and Italy in fighting the virus, enabling a third wave of the UK variant to build in the spring of 2021, forcing more painful lockdowns in France, Italy, and Germany.

Another piece of good news is that Operation Warp Speed taught the world not only that vaccines could be produced much faster than previously thought but also that the new mRNA technology used by Pfizer and Moderna enables production of much safer vaccines without weakened or dead virus in them.

Good Leaders and Politics Matter

The United States, Mexico, and Brazil failed to control SARS2 because their leaders failed: they attacked and undermined scientists, wouldn't wear masks and ridiculed people who did and refused to lock down their countries or reopened too early, creating amplification systems that fueled the surges that came after Christmas. India's prime minister Modi failed in his own way. In contrast, President Biden immediately appointed supremely competent scientists to run the CDC and advise him, getting 100 million Americans vaccinated in record time, and doing everything possible to get the virus under control.

In the United States and some parts of Europe, politicians were split over the most elementary actions necessary to fight pandemics, which is not a good sign. When every fact is politicized by politicians and the world sees each portraying itself as angels and the other side as devils, a country cannot unite against a virus. In the United States, part of the Republican Party opposes mask mandates, business lockdowns, and even vaccines.[29] Given such politicization, it seems that reservoirs of the virus and new hosts will exist in the United States for years to come. The growth of extremism everywhere hinders progress. Although most people adopt moderate positions in the middle, they often fail to see how that middle point can be altered by pushing the extremes on one side. To counter such extremism, Britain legalized censorship of false claims about vaccinations on social media.

India's Prime Minister Modi prematurely declared victory over Covid in March, just as dangerous new variants were spreading in India, including a new "double mutant" (B167) variant (unique to India). In April, he allowed the huge Kumbh Mela festival on the banks of the Ganges River, attracting a million Hindus, and he encouraged huge crowds at his rallies before the national election in April-May. As a result, Covid cases exploded in India, officially said to be 200,000 but probably far higher, with 3,000 deaths a day, hospitals overrun, patients dying from lack of oxygen and with only 1-2% of its population vaccinated.[30]

Brazil fared just as badly, with 3,000 deaths a day from its own variant and its Covid-denying President Bolsonaro warning that the Pfizer vaccine could turn recipients into crocodiles or bearded ladies, a remark featured in the *Hindu Times*.[31]

One Country Alone Cannot Fight Pandemics: The Need for Worldwide Cooperation

When it comes to dangerous infectious agents and pandemics, all humans face them together. Can we learn from the past? Can we learn that selfishness, tribalism, and vaccine nationalism do not create a viable future for the planet? Can we learn to cooperate to better and more quickly identify dangerous viruses, so that we can better control them?

We should stop the blame game. Without convincing evidence to the contrary, China appears to have not fully cooperated about the origins of SARS2 because it simply did not want to be blamed for being the origin of the virus. Similarly, American journalists adopted the name "Spanish flu" in 1918 to deflect attention from the origins of that flu in Kansas. Blame assumes that a country could have acted otherwise to prevent the emergence of the virus. That is unclear in the case of Covid-19, especially if the virus was transmitted from bats, which live in many different countries.

Vaccine nationalism helps rich nations but allows huge pockets of infection to fester around the globe, creating conditions for variants to emerge. If billions of people around the globe remain unvaccinated for the next few years, new variants will constantly emerge and stifle all hopes for herd immunity. Worldwide cooperation will be essential in defeating new variants, because "speed to detect" is critical for contact tracing, testing, and isolation.[32]

MORE PANDEMICS WILL COME

Pandemics are here to stay. The coronavirus that began in Wuhan will not be the last bad virus to appear, since the conditions that breed pandemics are not going away. First, global warming is real and will have profound effects on our lives. Second, we know that the world's population is exploding: in 2000, humans totaled over 6 billion; by 2022, they will total 8 billion, and by 2030, perhaps 10 billion.[33] More people create more crowding, more burning of wild habitat to make way for farms, and more close interaction of humans with wild animals—all conditions for creating new hybrid viruses that can jump from bats, pigs, chickens, and primates to humans. Bats are found on six continents. Chiropterologists to date have discovered over 1,200 species of them, and we know they carry many kinds of viruses. Because of antigenic drift and bat–human interactions, we know that hybrid viruses are always being formed. Birds also carry viruses, and migratory birds spread them across the globe.

And, finally, our world is growing increasingly connected. We now have just-in-time supply chains from distribution hubs in Louisville to finishing plants in Ohio to the giant container ships docking in California which deliver and bring manufactured goods from China, Vietnam, and Indonesia. These tight chains allow hybrid viruses to quickly spread.

WHAT WILL HAPPEN NEXT?

In the spring of 2021, a race unfolded across the globe, with countries trying to vaccinate as many people as possible while more infectious variants simultaneously spread. World leaders declared a war-time mentality and bioethicists debated measures to speed up vaccination. As this book goes to press, two big questions remain: who will win the race to vaccinate, and how long will existing vaccines work against SARS2 and its variants. Only time will tell.

NOTES

NOTES TO CHAPTER ONE

1 Laura Spinney, *Pale Rider: The Spanish Flu of 1918 and How It Changed the World* (New York: Hachette, 2017), 4.
2 Albert Camus, *The Plague*, translated by S. Gilbert (Penguin, 1960; originally published as *La Peste* [Paris: Gallimard, 1947]), 35.
3 The American press disguised its origins in Kansas and scapegoated Spain with a name that stuck. Ibid., 36.
4 Delia Owens, *Where the Crawdads Sing* (New York: Putnam's, 2018), 142–43.
5 Alfred Crosby, *American's Forgotten Pandemic: The Influenza of 1918*, 2nd ed. (1989; Cambridge: Cambridge University Press, 2003).
6 Laura Spinney, "What Does the Spanish Flu of 1918 Teach Us about Our Response to Pandemics?," National Public Radio, 18 December 2020.
7 John Barry, *The Great Influenza: The Story of the Deadliest Pandemic in History* (2004; New York: Penguin, 2018).
8 Stephen Mihm, "Philadelphia's Deadly Lesson," *Birmingham News*, 8 March 2020, A18.
9 Dan Barry and Caitlin Dickerson, "The Silent Killer of 1918: A Philadelphia Story," *New York Times*, 5 April 2020, 1, 12.
10 Barry, *The Great Influenza*.
11 Shannon Eblen, "Learning from Pandemics Past: Overshadowed by World War I, the Spanish Flu Gets a Closer Look," *New York Times*, 3 March 2020, F4.
12 Gina Kolata, *Flu: The Story of the Great Influenza Pandemic of 1918 and the Search for the Virus That Caused It* (New York: Atria Books, 2001).
13 *Proceedings of the National Academy of Science USA*, 104, no. 18 (2007): 7582–87.
14 Joshua Loomis, *Epidemics: The Impact of Germs and Their Power over Humanity* (New York: Prager, 2018), 201–02. Loomis's book also directed me to the reference above.
15 Ibid.
16 Rachel Bachman, "The Reason Football Played on in 1918," *Wall Street Journal*, 3 September 2020, A14.
17 Ibid.

18 Katherine Ann Porter, *Pale Horse, Pale Rider: Three Short Novels* (1939; New York: Harcourt Brace & Company, 1964), 163.

19 Michael Agresta, "The Great Texas Novel about the Spanish Flu," *Texas Monthly*, August 2020, 72–119.

20 Twila van Leer, "Flu Epidemic Hit Utah Hard in 1918, 1919," *Deseret News,* 28 March 1995.

21 Andre Noymer and Michel Garenne, "The 1918 Influenza Epidemic's Effects on Sex Differentials in Mortality in the United States," *Population Development Review* 26, no. 3 (2000): 565–81.

22 John Barry, quoted in "Year in Review," *USA Today*, 28 December 2020, 6A.

23 Spinney, "What Does the Spanish Flu of 1918 Teach Us?"

24 Loomis, *Epidemics*, 163–69.

25 Charles Rosenberg, *The Cholera Years* (Chicago: University of Chicago Press, 1962), 43.

26 Richard Conniff, "How Pandemics Change Us, What History Has Taught Us," *National Geographic*, August 2020, 58–59. Alas, initial efforts to solve the Great Stink made things worse. Because the miasmatic theory of cholera's transmission was the conventional wisdom, authorities aimed at preventing bad odors, so their solution was to dump more fecal material more quickly into rivers and creeks, thus completely contaminating the water supply. Thanks to G. Lynn Stephens for this insight.

27 Centers for Disease Control (CDC), "Cholera in Haiti," https://www.cdc.gov/cholera/haiti/index.html.

28 Jonathan M. Katz, "The U.N.'s Cholera Admission and What Comes Next," *New York Times Magazine*, 19 August 2016.

29 T. Mashe, "Highly Resistant Cholera Outbreak Strain in Zimbabwe," *New England Journal of Medicine* 383 (13 August 2020).

30 Barbara Tuchman, *A Distant Mirror: The Calamitous 14th Century* (1978; New York: Random House, 2014), 121.

31 Mary Douglas, *Purity and Danger: An Analysis of Concepts of Pollution and Taboo* (London: Routledge and Kegan Paul, 1966).

32 Philip Zeigler, *The Black Death* (New York: HarperCollins, 2009), 84–109.

33 Loomis, *Epidemics*, 37.

34 Gillian Brockell, "The African Roots of Inoculation in America: Saving Lives for Three Centuries," *Washington Post*, 15 December 2020.

35 Kent Sepkowitz, "The 1947 Smallpox Vaccination Campaign in New York City, Revisited," *Emerging Infectious Diseases* 10, no. 5 (2004): 960–61.

36 Quoting former CDC director Tom Frieden, *Wall Street Journal*, 5-6 December 2020, C1.

37 Howard Markel, quoted by Jenny Jarvive, "Ethical Dilemmas in the Age of Coronavirus: Whose Lives Should We Save?," *Los Angeles Times*, 19 March 2020.

NOTES TO CHAPTER TWO

1 Richard Preston, *The Hot Zone: The Terrifying True Story of the Origins of the Ebola Virus* (1994; New York, Anchor Books, 1995), 37–38.

2 Emma Goldberg, "Rollout of Vaccines Stirs Memories of a Scourge Conquered Decades Ago," *New York Times*, 31 December 2020, A8.

3 McGill Medicine cites 6,000 deaths and 27,000 cases nationwide (http://www.medicine.mcgill.ca/epidemiology/hanley/minimed/DiseaseMaryDobsonPolio.pdf and https://amhistory.si.edu/polio/americanepi/communities.htm). Almost all

studies cite *Epidemiological Studies of Poliomyelitis in New York City and the North-eastern United States during the Year 1916*, by Claude Hervey Lavinder, Allen Weir Freeman, and Wade Hampton Frost, for their polio statistics.

Thanks to historian-microbiologist Josh Loomis for helping me understand these figures, especially his comment that, "with the relatively primitive diagnostic tools available to them in 1916 and the fact that lots of infectious agents cause flu-like symptoms, I would bet that the vast majority of 'polio cases' reported then were actually cases of paralysis" (personal communication, 12 November 2020).

4 Loomis, *Epidemics*, 215.
5 CDC, "Polio Elimination in the United States," https://www.cdc.gov/polio/what-is-polio/polio-us.html.
6 Goldberg, "Rollout of Vaccines," A8.
7 Loomis, *Epidemics*, 222.
8 Saeed Shan and Betsy McKay, "Pandemic Delay Fuels Polio's Resurgence," *Wall Street Journal*, 10 February 2021, A1.
9 See Lawrence Wright, "The Plague Year," *The New Yorker*, 4 and 11 January 2021, 25.
10 CDC, "1968 Pandemic (H3N2 virus)," https://www.cdc.gov/flu/pandemic-resources/1968-pandemic.html.
11 Barbara J. Jester, Timothy M. Uyeki, and Daniel B. Jernigan, "Fifty Years of Influenza A(H3N2) following the Pandemic of 1968," *American Journal of Public Health* 110, no. 5 (2020): 669–76.
12 David M. Morrens, Peter Daszak, and Jeffery K. Taubenberger, "Escaping Pandora's Box: Another Novel Coronavirus," *New England Journal of Medicine* 382 (2 April 2020): 1293–95.
13 Preston, *The Hot Zone*.
14 CDC, "2014–2016 Ebola Outbreak in West Africa," https://www.cdc.gov/vhf/ebola/history/2014-2016-outbreak/index.html.
15 Ibid.
16 World Health Organization, "Swine Flu of 1976: Lessons of the Past," https://www.who.int/bulletin/volumes/87/6/09-040609/en/; Thomas Frieden, "The Three Key Hurdles for a Coronavirus Vaccine to Clear," *Wall Street Journal*, 31 July 2020.
17 Randy Shilts, *And the Band Played On: People, Politics and the AIDS Epidemic* (New York: St. Martin's Press, 1997).
18 Charles Stanley, quoted in Scripps Howard News Service, *Birmingham Post-Herald*, 21 January 1986.
19 Margaret Heckler, quoted in Shilts, *And the Band Played On*, 311.
20 Joseph Bove, quoted in ibid., 345.
21 Centers for Disease Control, "HIV by Group," https://www.cdc.gov/hiv/group/index.html.
22 Sarah Z. Hoffman, "HIV/AIDS in Cuba: A Model for Care or an Ethical Dilemma," *African Health Sciences* 4, no. 3 (2004): 208–09. See also Abdullah Saeed, "Why a Community of Punks Chose to Infect Themselves with HIV in Castro's Cuba," *Vice News*, 31 January 2017.
23 Robin McKie, "Scientists Trace 2002 Sars Virus to Colony of Cave-dwelling Bats in China," *The Guardian*, 9 December 2017.
24 Yongshi Yang et al., "The Deadly Coronaviruses: The 2003 SARS Pandemic and the 2020 Novel Coronavirus Epidemic in China," *Journal of Autoimmunology* 109 (2020).
25 CDC, "2009 H1N1 Pandemic Timeline," https://www.cdc.gov/flu/pandemic-resources/2009-pandemic-timeline.html.
26 Ibid.

27 Daniel DeNoon, "H1N1 Swine Flu No Worse Than Seasonal Flu," *WebMD*, 7 September 2010, https://www.webmd.com/cold-and-flu/news/20100907/h1n1-swine-flu-no-worse-than-seasonal-flu; "WHO and the Pandemic Flu 'Conspiracies,'" *British Medical Journal* 340 (2010): c2912.

28 CDC, "Narcolepsy following 2009 Pandemrix Influenza Vaccination in Europe," https://www.cdc.gov/vaccinesafety/concerns/history/narcolepsy-flu.html.

29 CDC, "Middle East Respiratory Syndrome (MERS)," https://www.cdc.gov/coronavirus/mers/index.html.

30 Pan Belleck et al., "Zika Virus Grew Deadlier with a Mutation, Study Suggests," *New York Times*, 29 September 2017, A9.

31 Kate Steiker-Ginzberg et al., "Xia's Ground Zero Still Struggling," *Asheville Citizen-Times*, 26 November 2017, B3.

32 Bara Vaida, "Zika Still a Threat in Puerto Rico, but Government Stopped Tracking It," *Covering Health: Association of Health Care Journalists*, 4 February 2019.

33 Jon Cohen, "Zika Has All but Disappeared in the Americas. Why?," *Science*, 16 August 2017.

34 Niall McCarthy, "How Many Americans Die from the Flu Each Year," *Statista*, 7 October 2020.

NOTES TO CHAPTER THREE

1 Lawrence Wright, *The End of October* (New York: Knopf, 2020).

2 "Mysteries of a Virus," *National Geographic*, February 2020, 46.

3 For a good synopsis of the competing theories, listen to Frank Sweeny, "COVID Commentaries. Episode 2: The Enemy Appears [Origins]," Straight Talk MD, https://podcasts.apple.com/us/podcast/covid-commentaries-episode-2-the-enemy-appears-origins/id1060256849?i=1000505892612.

4 Betsy McKay and Drew Hinshaw, "Virus Likely Spread Earlier Than Thought," *Wall Street Journal*, 20–21 February 2021, A8.

5 Peter Hessler, "The Sealed City," *The New Yorker*, 12 October 2020, 43.

6 Infectious proteins called "prions" also cause transmissible spongiform encephalopathies (TSEs), such as Creutzfeldt-Jakob Disease (CJD) in humans and Bovine Spongiform Encephalopathy (BSE) and Chronic Wasting Disease (CWD) in animals. See CDC, "Prion Diseases," https://www.cdc.gov/prions/index.html.

7 Loomis, *Epidemics*, 198.

8 James Glanz, Benedict Carey, and Hannah Beech, "Evidence Builds That an Early Mutation Made the Pandemic Harder to Stop," *New York Times*, 24 November 2020, A1.

9 Scott Engel Rasmussen, "Denmark to Cull Mink for Coronavirus Risk," *Wall Street Journal*, 6 November 2020; Larry Brilliant et al., "Herd Immunity Won't Save Us—But We Can Still Beat Covid-19," *Wall Street Journal*, 27–28 March 2021, C1.

10 Tracey Loew, "Oregon Mink Farm Discovers Covid-19 Outbreak," *USA Today*, 28 November 2020.

11 Jason Douglas, "Variant of Virus Identified in the U.K.," *Wall Street Journal*, 15 December 2020, A7.

12 Benjamin Mueller, "Scientists' Path to Variant Led through Genetic Sequence," *New York Times*, 17 January 2021, 4.

13 Kirsten Grieshaber and Sylvia Hui, "More EU Nations Ban Travel from UK, Fearing Virus Variant," ABC News, 20 December 2020.

14 Sheryl Gay Stolberg and Carl Zimmer, "Highly Contagious Variant Is Dominant in New Cases, C.D.C. Director Says," *New York Times*, 8 April 2021, A9.

15 CDC, "US COVID-19 Cases Caused by Variants," 18 January 2021; Helen Braswell, "New Coronavirus Variant Could Become Dominant Strain in March, CDC Warns," *Stat*, 15 January 2021; B. Pancivski, "Variants Outpace EU's Vaccine Rollout," *Wall Street Journal*, 17 February 2021, A9.

16 Apoora Mandavilli and Benjamin Mueller, "Rising Variants Imperil Return to Normal Life," *New York Times*, 4 April 2021, A1.

17 "New Virus Variants Raise Alarms," *The Week*, 12 February 2021, 4.

18 Mandavilli and Mueller, "Rising Variants," 6.

19 Daniel Michaels and Jason Douglas, "Countries Ban Travel from U.K. in Race to Block New Covid-19 Strain," *Wall Street Journal*, 20 December 2020.

20 "Canada Ski Resort Linked to Largest Outbreak of P1 Covid Variant outside Brazil," *The Guardian*, 11 April 2021.

21 Jill Lawless, *Birmingham News*, 14 January 2021, A6.

22 Josh Holder et al., "Deadlier, More Contagious Variants Tearing across Europe Show Virus Remains a Threat," *New York Times*, 11 April 2021, A8.

23 CDC, "SARS-CoV-2 Variant Classifications and Definitions," https://www.cdc.gov/ coronavirus/2019-ncov/cases-updates/variant-surveillance/variant-info.html.

24 William Shaffer, quoted by Pam Belluck, "What Exactly Does This Virus Do in the Body?," *New York Times*, 17 March 2020, D7.

25 Ibid.

26 Steven Reinberg, "More Symptoms of Coronavirus: COVID Toes, Skin Rashes," *Medical Press*, 4 May 2020.

27 Jan Hoffman, "Smokers and Vapers May Be at Greater Risk of Getting Coronavirus," *New York Times*, 9 April 2020.

28 Smriti Mallapaty, "The Coronavirus Is Most Deadly If You Are Older and Male," *Nature*, 28 August 2020.

29 Ed Yong, "COVID Can Last for Several Months," *The Atlantic*, 15 June 2020.

30 "Proning COVID Patients Reduces Need for Ventilator," *Columbia University Medical Center News*, 2 July 2020.

31 Daniela Lamas, "I'm on the Front Lines. I Have No Plan for This," *New York Times*, 24 March 2020; Daniela Lamas, "To My Patients' Family Members, My Apologies," *New York Times*, 20 May 2020.

32 See Kolata, *Flu*.

33 David Fajenbaum and Carl June, "Cytokine Storm," *New England Journal of Medicine* 383 (3 December 2020).

34 Matt Windsor, "Cytokine Storm Treatment for Coronavirus Patients Is Focus of First-in-US Study," *UAB Reporter*, 29 April 2020.

35 Loomis, *Epidemics*, 195.

36 Jamie Weisman, *As I Live and Breathe: Notes of a Patient-Doctor* (New York: Farrar, Straus and Giroux, 2002), 10.

37 CDC, "Risk of Covid-19 Infection, Hospitalization, and Deaths by Race/Ethnicity," https://www.cdc.gov/coronavirus/2019-ncov/covid-data/investigations-discovery/ hospitalization-death-by-race-ethnicity.html.

38 Neil M. Ferguson et al., "Report 9: Impact of Non-Pharmaceutical Interventions (NPIs) to Reduce COVID-19 Mortality and Healthcare Demand," Imperial College London, 16 March 2020, https://www.imperial.ac.uk/mrc-global-infectious-disease-analysis/ covid-19/report-9-impact-of-npis-on-covid-19/.

39 Brianna Abbott and Jason Douglas, "How Deadly Is COVID? Researchers Are Getting Closer to an Answer," *Wall Street Journal*, 21 July 2020.

40 Ibid.

41 The CDC cites 675,000 deaths in the United States from the Spanish flu, rather than half a million (CDC, "1918 Pandemic (H1N1 Virus)," https://www.cdc.gov/flu/pandemic-resources/1918-pandemic-h1n1.html). Since the US population in 1918 was about 103.2 million, this would mean around 0.65 percent of the population died. The US population is currently around 331 million, so the 2020 Covid equivalent would then be around 2.2 million deaths. Some sources use 0.5 percent instead of 0.65 percent; using 0.5 percent would give a Covid equivalent of around 1.66 million American deaths.

42 CDC, "Covid Mortality Overview," https://www.cdc.gov/nchs/covid19/mortality-overview.htm.

43 Mike Ives et al., "Virus Casualties Pass 3 Million as Hot Spots Emerge Anew," *New York Times*, 18 April 2021, 4.

44 Kaiser Health News, "Lost on the Frontline," https://www.theguardian.com/us-news/ng-interactive/2020/aug/11/lost-on-the-frontline-covid-19-coronavirus-us-health-care-workers-deaths-database. For its prize, see "Guardian US and Kaiser Health News Win Batten Medal for 'Lost on the Frontline,'" *The Guardian*, 5 April 2021.

45 Jordan Kisner, "The Committee on Life and Death," *The Atlantic*, January–February 2021, 40.

46 Daniel B. Kramer, Bernard Lo, and Neal W. Dickert, "CPR in the Covid-19 Era: An Ethical Framework," *New England Journal of Medicine* 383 (9 July 2020).

47 Ibid. Note that "crisis standards of care" is a technical phrase in some states that, when invoked by a governor, may give staff some immunity from lawsuits and allow formal triage. During the Covid pandemic, almost no governors declared such standards.

48 CDC, "Health Department-Reported Cases of Multisystem Inflammatory Syndrome in Children (MIS-C) in the United States," https://www.cdc.gov/mis-c/cases/index.html.

49 Pam Belluck, "Mysterious Malady Hits the Asymptomatic Young," *New York Times*, 7 April 2021, A6.

50 Linsey Marr, "Yes, the Coronavirus Is in the Air," *New York Times*, 3 August 2020, A21.

51 CDC, "Absence of Apparent Transmission of SARS-CoV-2 from Two Stylists after Exposure at a Hair Salon with a Universal Face Covering Policy—Springfield, Missouri, May 2020," *Morbidity and Mortality Weekly Report* 69, no. 28 (17 July 2020): 930–32.

52 Monica Gandhi, interviewed by Ailsa Chang, "Growing Body of Evidence Suggests Masks Protect Those Wearing Them, Too," *National Public Radio*, 20 July 2020.

53 Emily Anthies, "Chance of Catching Covid from Surfaces Is Low," *New York Times*, 9 April 2021, A4.

54 Emily Anthies, "Air Sampler Searches for Covid-19 Particles, Then Acts as a Captor," *New York Times*, 25 March 2021, A7.

55 Apoorva Mandavilli, "'A Smoking Gun': Infectious Coronavirus Retrieved from Hospital Air," *New York Times*, 11 August 2020.

56 Environmental Protection Agency, "Air Cleaners, HVAC Filters, and Coronavirus (COVID-19)," https://www.epa.gov/coronavirus/air-cleaners-hvac-filters-and-coronavirus-covid-19.

57 Mike Baker, "What Will Winter Bring?," *New York Times*, 21 October 2020.

58 Michael Wines and Amy Harmon, "Feb. Superspreader Kept Spreading, Infecting as Many as 300,000 by Oct.," *New York Times*, 11 December 2020; Karen Weintraub,

"Study Eyes Outbreaks at Super-Spreading Events," *USA Today*, 27 August 2020.

59 Emily Woodruff, "1 COVID Carrier, 50,000 Infections," *Time-Picayune/New Orleans Advocate*, 12 February 2021.

60 Mark Walter and Jack Healy, "A Motorcycle Rally in a Pandemic? 'We Kind of Knew What Was Going to Happen,'" *New York Times*, 7 November 2020.

61 Apoorva Mandavilli, "Children May Carry the Virus at High Levels," *New York Times*, 31 July 2020, A4.

62 Centers for Disease Control, "SARS-CoV-2 Transmission and Infection among Attendees of an Overnight Camp—Georgia, June 2020," https://www.cdc.gov/mmwr/volumes/69/wr/mm6931e1.htm.

63 Ibid.

64 Jared Hopkins, "Pfizer Shot Effective after Six Months," *Wall Street Journal*, 2 April 2021, A6.

65 Gina Kolata, "Vaccine Study Confirms Effectiveness in Real World," *New York Times*, 29 March 2021, A3.

66 Andrew Joseph, "First COVID Reinfection Documented in Hong Kong, Researchers Say," *STAT NEWs*, 24 August 2020.

67 Joshua Robinson, "The Cyclist Who Caught Covid-19 Twice," *Wall Street Journal*, 3 December 2020, A14; "Suspected Cases of COVID-19 Reinfection," *COVID-19 Reinfection Tracker*, BNO News.

68 Pam Belluck, "He Was Hospitalized for Covid-19, Then Again, and Again," *New York Times*, 30 December 2020.

69 CDC, "Characteristics of Hospitalized COVID-19 Patients Discharged and Experiencing Same-Hospital Readmission—United States, Mar.–Aug. 2020," *Morbidity and Mortality Weekly Report* 69, no. 45 (13 November 2020): 1695–99.

70 Anthony Fauci, "Fauci to Medscape: 'We're All in It Together and We're Gonna Get through It,'" *Medscape*, 17 July 2020.

71 Fiona Lowenstein, "A Long Road to Recovery," *New York Times*, 1 April 2020.

72 Adrianna Rodriquez, "Chronic COVID Can Last Miserable Months," *USA Today*, 22 June 2020, D1.

73 Katarina Zimmer, "Could COVID-19 Trigger Chronic Disease in Some People?" *The Scientist*, 17 July 2020.

74 See https://www.survivorcorps.com.

75 Pam Belluck, "6 Months Later, Survivors Plagued by Problems," *New York Times*, 14 January 2021.

76 Ed Yong, "The Covid-19 Manhattan Project," *The Atlantic*, January–February 2021, 53.

77 Fauci, "Fauci to Medscape."

78 Melinda Wenner Moyer, "Can COVID Damage the Brain?" *New York Times*, 29 June 2020; Grace Hauck, "COVID in the Brain?" *USA Today*, 30 June 2020.

79 Sally Robertson, "COVID May Damage the Central Nervous System," *News-Medical.net*, 22 May 2020; Lois Parshley, "How Long Does the Coronavirus Last Inside the Body?," *National Geographic*, 3 June 2020.

80 Pam Belluck, "Beating Covid, Only to Be Left with Brain Fog," *New York Times*, 12 October 2020, A1, A6.

81 Adrianna Rodriquez, "Study: Heart Damage Found in Virus Patients Months after Recovery," *USA Today*, 30 July 2020.

82 Inbal Benhar et al., "The Privileged Immunity of Immune Privileged Organs: The Case of the Eye." *Frontiers in Immunology*, Frontiers Research Foundation, 21 September 2012.

83 James Hamblin, "The Mysterious Link between COVID-19 and Sleep," *The Atlantic*, 21 December 2020.

84 Pam Belluck, "For Some, Psychosis Follows Covid," *New York Times*, 28 December 2020, D1.

85 Jeremy Devine, "The Dubious Origins of Long Covid," *Wall Street Journal*, 23 March 2021, A15.

86 Yochai Re'em, "The Science Behind 'Long Covid' and the Dubious Desire to Wish It Away," *Wall Street Journal*, 30 March 2021, A16.

NOTES TO CHAPTER FOUR

1 William Cummings, "Poll: 57% of GOP Says COVID-19 Deaths Acceptable," *USA Today*, 25 August 2020.

2 Morgan Hines, "CDC Data: Cruises Amplify, Scatter COVID Spread," *USA Today*, 22 July 2020, D4.

3 William *Feuer,* "CDC Says Coronavirus RNA Found in Princess Cruise Ship Cabins up to 17 Days after Passengers Left," *CNBC*, 28 March 2020.

4 The Yomiuri Shimbun, "Japan Paid 94% of Medical Costs for Foreign Passengers on Coronavirus-Hit Cruise Ship," *Japan News*, 12 November 2020.

5 Peer Hessler, "The Sealed City," *New Yorker*, 12 October 2020, 40.

6 COVID Dashboard of Johns Hopkins University, https://coronavirus.jhu.edu/map.html.

7 "Great Barrington Declaration," https://gbdeclaration.org/.

8 Ibid.

9 Siobhan Roberts, "Beating the Pandemic with a Swiss Cheese Defense," *New York Times*, 7 December 2020.

10 Yaryna Serkez, "A 20 Percent Shutdown Could Be Enough," *New York Times*, 17 December 2020, A23.

11 Eduardo Porter, "Selective Closures Would Better Halt the Virus, Researchers Say," *New York Times*, 6 June 2020.

12 Philippe Lemoine, "The Lockdowns Weren't Worth It," *Wall Street Journal*, 1 March 2021, A15.

13 ABC News, 13 August 2020.

14 Thomas Harr, quoted by Peter Goodman, "Sweden Has Become the World's Cautionary Tale," *New York Times*, 7 July 2020, updated 15 July 2020.

15 25 Swedish doctors and scientists, "Sweden Hoped Herd Immunity Would Curb COVID-19. Don't Do What We Did. It's Not Working," *USA Today*, 21 July 2020.

16 Goodman, "Sweden Has Become the World's Cautionary Tale."

17 Bojan Pacevski, "Holdout Sweden Ends Its Covid-19 Experiment," *Wall Street Journal*, 7 December 2020; Drew Hinshaw, "Sweden's Voluntary Covid-10 Measures Come Under Fire," *Wall Street Journal*, 17 December 2020.

18 Jacob Ausubel, "Populations Skew Older in Countries Hard Hit by Covid," *Pew Research Center*, 22 April 2020.

19 Alex de Waal and Paul Richards, "Coronavirus: Why Lockdowns May Not Be the Answer in Africa," *BBC News*, 14 April 2020; Benjamin Smart, Alex Broadbent, and Herkulaas Combrink, "Lockdown Didn't Work in South Africa: Why It Shouldn't Happen Again," *The Conversation*, 15 October 2020.

20 "Who Lives Longest? Top 20 Nations in Life Expectancy," *CBS News*, 29 November 2018.

21 Ausubel, "Populations Skew Older."
22 Johns Hopkins COVID Dashboard.
23 Siddhartha Mukherjee, "The Covid Conundrum," *New Yorker*, 1 March 2021, 19.
24 Smart et al., "Lockdown Didn't Work in South Africa."
25 Jacob Horowitz, "The Lessons of a Global Pariah that Turned into a Containment Success Story," *New York Times*, 1 August 2020, A7.
26 Melissa Eddy, "Merkel Announces Strict Lockdown Over Holidays," *New York Times*, 14 December 2020, A7.
27 Melissa Eddy, "Traveling to Germany? A Free COVID Test Awaits," *New York Times*, 6 August 2020, A8.
28 International Monetary Fund, "Kurzarbeit: Germany's Short-Time Work Benefit," 15 June 2020.
29 Ruchir Sharma, "Not Every Nation Is Ready for the Post-COVID Era," *New York Times*, 19 July 2020.
30 Peter S. Goodman, Liz Alderman, and Jack Ewing, "Europe Flashes Signs of Hope Amid a Plunge," *New York Times*, 1 August 2020, A1.
31 Ruth Bender, "Weary Europe Despairs Over Virus," *Wall Street Journal*, 24 March 2021, A18.
32 HyunJung Kim, "South Korea Learned Its Successful COVID Strategy from a Previous Coronavirus Outbreak: MERS," *Bulletin of the Atomic Scientists*, 20 March 2020.
33 Keren Landman, "What We Can Learn from South Korea's Coronavirus Response," *Elemental*, 1 June 2020.
34 Jeremy Howard et al., "An Evidence Review of Face Masks against COVID-19," *Proceedings of the National Academy of Sciences* 118, no. 4 (26 January 2021).
35 C. Taylor, "How New Zealand's 'Eliminate' Strategy Brought New Coronavirus Cases Down to Zero," *CNBC.com*, 5 May 2020.
36 Ibid.
37 Ministry of Health, "COVID: Elimination Strategy for Aotearoa New Zealand," 8 May 2020, https://www.health.govt.nz/our-work/diseases-and-conditions/covid-19-novel-coronavirus/covid-19-response-planning/covid-19-elimination-strategy-aotearoa-new-zealand.
38 T. Coughlan, "Coronavirus: The Government's COVID Lockdown Measures Have Overwhelming Public Support, According to A Poll," *Stuff*, 23 April 2020.
39 Ministry of Health, "COVID."
40 Damien Cave, "A Lesson from Australia: One Positive Covid-19 Test and a City Is Locked Down," *New York Times*, 3 February 2021.
41 Pam Tanowitz, "Fly to Australia. Lock Down. And, Yes, Work," *New York Times*, 4 April 2021, A8.
42 Melanie Warner, "How Hawaii Became a Rare COVID Success Story," *Politico*, 19 June 2020.
43 Elizabeth Kolbert, "How Iceland Beat the Coronavirus," *New Yorker*, 8/15 June 2020.
44 Daniel F. Gudbjartsson et al., "Spread of SARS-CoV-2 in the Icelandic Population," *New England Journal of Medicine* 382 (11 June 2020): 2302–15.
45 "COVID: First Results of the Voluntary Screening in Iceland," *Nordic Life Science*, 23 March 2020.
46 Kolbert, "How Iceland Beat the Coronavirus."
47 F. Norrestad, "Cumulative Number of Coronavirus (COVID) Cases in Iceland since Feb. 2020 (as of July 27, 2020)," Statista.com, 29 July 2020.
48 "Special Committee on the COVID Pandemic," House of Commons, 29 April 2020.

49 Evan Dyer, "COVID Taught Canada a Costly Lesson—That Early Border Closures Can Work," *CBC News*, 22 June 2020.

50 Ibid.

51 Rachel Aiello, "Canada-U.S. Border Likely to Remain Closed for Weeks, PM Says in Imposing Tougher Quarantine Rules," *CTV News*, 14 April 2020.

52 Canada, "Coronavirus Disease (COVID): Outbreak Update," https://www.canada.ca/en/public-health/services/diseases/coronavirus-disease-covid-19.html.

53 Sandrine Rastello and Kait Bolongaro, "Pfizer Delay Compounds Canada's Problems in Vaccine Campaign," *Bloomberg News*, 21 January 2021.

54 Justin Rowlatt, "Why India Wiped out 88% of Its Cash Overnight," *BBC News*, 14 November 2016.

55 Jeffrey Gettleman et al., "The Virus Trains: How Lockdown Chaos Spread COVID-19 across India," *New York Times*, 15 December 2020, A1; updated 2 February 2021.

56 Virhuti Agarawal and Eric Bellman, "India's Economy Shrinks at Record Pace," *Wall Street Journal*, 1 September 2020, A16.

57 Karan Deep Singh, "Lockdown and Despair Sow Death in Rural India," *New York Times*, 8 September 2020, A1, A6.

58 Gettleman et al., "Virus Trains."

59 Emily Schmall, "Indian Farmers' Protests Spread, in Challenge to Modi," *New York Times*, 4 December 2020.

60 Luciana Magalhaes and Kejal Vyas, "Brazil's COVID Deaths Top 100,000," *Wall Street Journal*, 10 August 2020, A7.

61 Juan Montes and Vibhuti Agarwal, "Developing Nations Face Long Pandemic," *Wall Street Journal*, 13 August 2020, A16.

62 Donald Trump, quoted by Michael Shear et al., "Trump's Focus as the Pandemic Raged," *New York Times*, 31 December 2020; updated 13 January 2021.

63 Johns Hopkins COVID Dashboard.

64 Gus Garcia-Roberts, Erin Mansfield, and Caroline Anders, "It May Not Have Started Here, but the Novel Coronavirus Became a US Tragedy," *USA Today*, 10 December 2020; updated 26 January 2021: Gus Garcia-Roberts et al., "How the US Failed to Meet the Challenge of Covid 19," *USA Today*, 11 December 2020.

65 Khrysgiana Pineda, "Reviewing Thousands of Deaths, Millions of Cases," *USA Today*, 24 July 2020, A4. The United States has many dual citizens who hold certificates in another country. It would have been difficult to ban such citizens from returning home (although China and Japan did just that).

66 M. Holshue et al., "First Case of 2019 Novel Coronavirus in the United States," *New England Journal of Medicine* 382 (5 March 2020): 929–36.

67 James Gorman, "Virus May Have Reached U.S. in Dec., Not Jan.," *New York Times*, 1 December 2020.

68 Khrysgiana Pineda, "Reviewing Thousands of Deaths, Millions of Cases," *USA Today*, 24 July 2020, A4.

69 Donald McNeil, "Former Head of Health Agency Urges States to Standardize Data," *New York Times*, 23 July 2020.

70 Ibid.

71 Tim Murphy, "Have Known Him a Long Time," *The BodyPro*, 20 March 2020.

72 Michael Specter, "How Fauci Became America's Doctor," *New Yorker*, 13 April 2020.

73 Paul Offit, quoted from podcast, *Straight Talk, MD*, Episode #131, "Overkill: When Modern Medicine Goes Too Far with Paul Offit," http://straighttalkmd.com/podcast/overkill/.

74 Warren Cornwall, "Just 50% of Americans Plan to Get a COVID Vaccine. Here's How to Win Over the Rest," *Science*, 30 June 2020.

75 Editorial, *New England Journal of Medicine* 384 (20 October 2020): 576.

76 Allysisa Finley, "Vindication for Ron DeSantis," *Wall Street Journal*, 6–7 March 2021.

NOTES TO CHAPTER FIVE

1 Jenny Jarvie, "Ethical Dilemmas in the Age of Coronavirus: Whose Lives Should We Save?" *Los Angeles Times*, 19 March 2020.

2 Lisa Rosenbaum, "Facing Covid-19 in Italy—Ethics, Logistics, and Therapeutics on the Epidemic's Front Line," *New England Journal of Medicine* 382 (18 March 2020): 1873–75.

3 William McAskill, *Doing Good Better: Effective Altruism* (New York: Avery, 2015).

4 Hiroyuki Nakao et al., "A Review of the History of the Origin of Triage from a Disaster Medicine Perspective," *Acute Medicine and Surgery* 4, no. 4 (4 October 2017): 379–84.

5 Robert Seinbrook, "The AIDS Epidemic: A Progress Report from Mexico City," *New England Journal of Medicine* 359, no. 9 (28 August 2008): 886.

6 Munyaradzi Makoni, "Tanzania Refuses COVID-19 Vaccines," *The Lancet* 397 (13 February 2021).

7 See Gregory Pence, *Medical Ethics: Accounts of Ground-Breaking Cases*, 9th ed. (New York: McGraw-Hill, 2020), 279.

8 Elizabeth Anscombe, "Mr. Truman's Degree" (Oxford: Oxonian Press, 1956).

9 John Rawls, *A Theory of Justice* (Cambridge, MA: Belknap Press of Harvard University, 1971).

10 So says Maximus in the 2000 movie *Gladiator,* presumably representing the ideas of second-century Roman philosopher Marcus Aurelius.

11 Jacob Bunge, "U.S. Regulators Fine Pork Giant Smithfield over Covid Outbreak," *Wall Street Journal*, 10 September 2020.

12 Alasdair MacIntyre, *A Short History of Ethics* (New York: Macmillan, 1966).

13 Gregory Pence, "The God Committee," Chapter 11, *Medical Ethics*, 9th ed. (New York: McGraw-Hill, 2020).

14 Nicholas Rescher, "The Allocation of Exotic Lifesaving Therapy," *Ethics* 79 (April 1969).

15 Ezekiel J. Emanuel et al., "Fair Allocation of Scarce Medical Resources in the Time of Covid," *New England Journal of Medicine* 382 (21 May 2020): 2049–55.

16 Doug White, "Allocation of Scarce Critical Care Resources during a Public Health Emergency," University of Pittsburgh Medical Center, 15 April 2020.

17 Ronald Buerk, "Japan Pensioners Volunteer to Tackle Nuclear Crisis," *BBC News*, 31 May 2011

18 Paula Span, "Should Youth Come First in Coronavirus Care?" *New York Times*, 4 August 2020, D3.

19 John Hardwig, "Is There a Duty to Die?," *Hastings Center Report* 27, no. 2 (March–April 1997): 34–42.

20 Larry R. Churchill, "On Being an Elder in a Pandemic," *New York Times*, 13 April 2020; Franklin G. Miller, "Why I Support Age-Related Rationing of Ventilators for Covid Patients," *Hastings Bioethics Forum*, 9 April 2020.

21 J.O. Urmson, "Saints and Heroes," in *Twentieth-Century Ethical Theory*, ed. Steven M. Cahn and Joram G. Haber (Englewood Cliffs, NJ: Prentice-Hall, 1995).

22 Johnny Kampis, "Alabama's Pandemic Emergency Plan Discriminates against People with Disabilities," *Tuscaloosa News*, 31 March 2020.

23 Joseph Fins, "Disabusing the Disability Critique of the New York State Task Force Report on Ventilator Allocation," *Hastings Bioethics Forum*, 1 April 2020.

24 See B. Huberman et al., "Phases of a Pandemic Surge: The Experience of an Ethics Service in New York City during Covid-19," *Journal of Clinical Ethics* 31, no. 3 (2020), 219–27; Joseph Fins and K. Prager, "The Covid-19 Crisis and Clinical Ethics in New York City," *Journal of Clinical Ethics* 31, no. 3 (2020): 228–32.

25 Katherine Wu, "Combat Fatigue," *New York Times*, 1 December 2020, D5.

26 Ibid.

27 Jordan Kisner, "The Committee on Life and Death," *The Atlantic*, January–February 2021, 40.

NOTES TO CHAPTER SIX

1 See Gregory Pence, "Ethical Issues in First-Time Organ Surgeries," in *Medical Ethics*, 240–66.

2 Pasteur's notebooks suggest he borrowed a famous cure for anthrax from that of his assistant, veterinary surgeon Jean Toussaint, who died at age 43, making him unable to press his claims.

3 David Quammen, "How Viruses Shape Our World," *National Geographic*, February 2021, 57.

4 Paul Offit, *Vaccinated: One Man's Quest to Defeat the World's Greatest Diseases* (New York: HarperCollins, 2005).

5 CDC, "Vaccine Safety: Overview, History, and How the Safety Process Works," https://www.cdc.gov/vaccinesafety/ensuringsafety/history/index.html.

6 CDC, "Understanding mRNA COVID-19 Vaccines," https://www.cdc.gov/coronavirus/2019-ncov/vaccines/different-vaccines/mrna.html.

7 John Hammontree, "When Can We Expect a Vaccine? Is It Safe to Go to School? UAB's Dr. Jeanne Marrazzo Talks about the Biggest COVID Questions," *Birmingham News*, 23 July 2020.

8 Mike Zimmerman, "A Vaccine Made for Those 50-Plus?" *AARP Bulletin*, August 2020, 18.

9 Jared Hopkins, "Vaccine Efforts Turn to Seniors," *Wall Street Journal*, 17 October 2020.

10 Ibid.

11 Ibid.

12 CDC, "Vaccine Safety."

13 CDC, "Vaccine Adverse Event Reporting System (VAERS)," https://www.cdc.gov/vaccinesafety/ensuringsafety/monitoring/vaers/index.html.

14 Quoted by Brian Mueller, "Criticisms of Human Challenge Studies," *New York Times*, 20 October 2020.

15 Joe Palca, "Britain Moves toward Ethically Controversial COVID-19 Vaccine Trial," *National Public Radio*, 21 October 2020.

16 Richard Yetter Chappell and Peter Singer, "Pandemic Ethics: The Case for Experiments on Human Volunteers," *Washington Post*, 27 April 2020.

17 One Day Sooner, https://www.1daysooner.org/.

18 Chappell and Singer, "Pandemic Ethics."

19 https://1daysooner.org/openletter.

20 Nir Eyal et al., "Human Challenge Studies to Accelerate Coronavirus Vaccine Licen-sure," *Journal of Infectious Disease* 221, no. 11 (11 May 2020): 1752–56.

21 Seema Sha, Holly Lynch, and Franklin Miller, "Before Deliberately Infecting People with Coronavirus, Be Sure It's Worth It," *New York Times*, 2 June 2020.

22 This point was made in an interview with Professor Melissa Nolan, an infectious disease expert at the University of South Carolina on the BBC News, 1 August 2020.

23 World Health Organization, "Dengue and Severe Dengue," https://www.who.int/news-room/fact-sheets/detail/dengue-and-severe-dengue.

24 Lisa Rosenbaum, "Trolleyology and the Dengue Vaccine Dilemma," *New England Journal of Medicine* 379 (26 July 2018): 305–07.

25 See Immanuel Kant, *The Metaphysical Principles of Virtue*, trans. James Ellington (Indianapolis: Bobbs-Merrill, 1965), 64; *Foundations of the Metaphysics of Morals*, trans. Lewis White Beck (Indianapolis: Bobbs-Merrill, 1965), 47.

26 "Covid-19: Human Challenge Studies Will See People Purposefully Infected with Virus," *British Medical Journal* 37 (22 October 2020).

27 Benjamin Mueller, "Britain Approves Study that Will Deliberately Infect Volunteers with the Virus," *New York Times*, 18 February 2021, A6.

28 M.J. Glesby and D.R. Hoover, "Survivor Treatment Selection Bias in Observational Studies: Examples from the AIDS Literature," *Annals of Internal Medicine* 124 (1 June 1996): 1003.

29 Katie Thomas, "Quest for Vaccine Was a Race, Availability Could Be a Crawl," *New York Times*, 18 November 2020, A1.

30 Interview with David Agus, *CBS Morning Show*, 15 December 2020.

31 Benjamin Mueller, "Allies Spar, in a Case of 'Vaccine Nationalism,'" *New York Times*, 4 December 2020.

32 Jason Douglas and Stephen Fidler, "U.K.'s NHS Faces a Vaccine Test," *Wall Street Journal*, 4 December 2020.

33 Sharon LaFraniere et al., "Scientists Fret as White House Rushes Vaccine," *New York Times*, 3 August 2020, A1.

34 Ibid.

35 Arthur Kramer, "Russia Sets Mass Vaccination for Oct. after Shortened Trial," *New York Times*, 2 August 2020.

NOTES TO CHAPTER SEVEN

1 Katie Thomas, "New Pfizer Results: Coronavirus Vaccine Is Safe and 95% Effective," *New York Times*, 18 November 2020.

2 Carl Zimmer, "What Does It Mean if 2 Companies Report 95% Efficacy Rates?" *New York Times*, 21 November 2020, A10.

3 Catherine Porter, "First Doses in Canada Prompt Tears of Relief," *New York Times*, 15 December 2020.

4 Carolyn Bormann, "Countdown to Immunity," *New Yorker*, 14 December 2020, 28.

5 Georgi Kantchev, "Russia Gets a Dose of Reality on Vaccines," *New York Times*, 11 December 2020.

6 Prashant Yadav of the Global Center for International Development, quoted by Eliza-beth Weise and K. Weinbraub, "Pfizer Plants across the Country," *USA Today*, 9 Feb-ruary 2021, D1.

7 Elisabeth Weise, "50 States, 50 Plans," *USA Today*, 8 December 2020, A1.

8 Amanda Coletta, "Canada Has Secured More Vaccine Doses Per Capita Than Anyone Else, but It's Been Slow to Administer Them," *Washington Post*, 15 January 2021.

9   Douglas Starr, *Blood: An Epic History of Medicine and Commerce* (New York: Harper, 2000).

10 Melanie Evans, "Hospitals Race to Prioritize Shots for Staffers," *Wall Street Journal*, 7 December 2020.

11 New York's Northwell Health ranked its 74,000 workers across 23 hospitals by risk of catching the virus on the job. Similarly, Minnesota's Allina Health system prioritized those among its 15,000 employees who interacted directly with coronavirus patients. Advocate Aurora Health Inc in Illinois and Wisconsin identified workers at greatest risk of severe illness in its 26 hospitals and clinics.

12 Brad Brooks, "Texas Doctors in Rural Hotspots Left Out in Cold on Vaccine," *ABC News/Reuters*, 18 December 2020; Ariel Hart et al., "Questions Arise in Vaccine Distribution as Georgia Tops 500,000 COVID-19 Cases," *Atlanta-Journal Constitution*, 18 December 2020; "Despite Some of the Highest Rates of Covid Cases, Two Western Maryland Counties Won't Receive Any of First-Round Vaccines," *Baltimore Sun*, 20 December 2020.

13 The CDC's data tracker cites 274,909 cases and 917 deaths among health-care personnel. These data were from early December 2020 but aren't entirely accurate because health-care personnel status and death status weren't available for all the people that the CDC collected data from. The *Guardian* and *Kaiser Health News* have a collaborative database that cites over 3,000 health-care worker deaths. These data are based on journalists' searches through websites and memorial pages. The Centers for Medicare & Medicaid Services website reports 322,690 cases and 1,162 deaths among nursing-home staff. These data are reported by nursing homes to the CDC's NHSN system and were current as of November 29, 2020. Also see Chapter 3, note 44.

14 Mo Lingli, *CBS National News*, 18 December 2020.

15 Mike Zaveri, "Who Gets Vaccine Next?" *New York Times*, 21 December 2020, A1.

16 Scott Gottlieb, "Who'll Get the Covid Vaccine First?" *Wall Street Journal*, 6 December 2020.

17 Paul Peterson, "Vaccination by Age Is the Way to Go," *New York Times*, 13 January 2021, A15.

18 Thomas Frieden and Christopher Lee, "Identifying and Interrupting Superspreader Events: Implications for Control of Severe Acute Respiratory Syndrome SARS2," *Emerging Infectious Diseases* 26, no. 6 (June 2020).

19 Tomas Philipson, "No Need to Sweat Covid Vaccination Rates," *Wall Street Journal*, 24 September 2020, A19.

20 Aaron Strong and Jonathan Welborn, "Teachers Should Get the Covid Vaccine First," *New York Times*, 20 November 2020, A15.

21 Adam Tamburin, "Meharry Leader Says Medical College 'Somehow' Didn't Get First Wave of Covid Vaccines," *The Tennessean*, 22 December 2020.

22 Rebecca Robbins, "Vaccine's Slow Path to Nursing Homes," *New York Times*, 18 January 2021.

23 Abby Goodnough and Jan Hoffman, "Officials Agonize over Recipients of First Vaccines," *New York Times*, 6 December 2020, A1, A6.

24 Sarah Krouse and Jacob Bunger, "Industries Vie for Vaccine Priority," *Wall Street Journal*, 12–13 December 2020, A6.

25 Ibid.

26 John Ingold, "Colorado's Governor Says Prisoners Won't Be Prioritized for a Coronavirus Vaccine. A State Plan Outlines Otherwise," *Colorado Sun*, 2 December 2020.

27 Keaton Ross, "Oklahoma Inmates and Corrections Staff Will Wait on Covid-19 Vaccine," *Oklahoma Watch*, 23 December 2020.

28 Oklahoma State Department of Health, COVID-19 Vaccine Priority Population Framework for Oklahoma, https://oklahoma.gov/content/dam/ok/en/covid19/documents/vaccine/COVID-19%20Vaccine%20Priority%20Population%20Framework%20for%20Oklahoma%20-%2012-10-20.pdf.

29 Glenn Howatt, "Minnesota Health Care Providers Question COVID-19 Vaccine Allocations," *(Minneapolis) Star Tribune*, 23 December, 2020.

30 Catherine E. Shoichet, "Covid-19 Is Taking a Devastating Toll on Filipino American Nurses," CNN, 24 November 2020.

31 Paul Fain, "Syracuse to Test Sewage for Coronavirus," *Inside Higher Education*, 5 June 2020.

32 Carl Zimmer and Noah Wieland, "Should Volunteers Who Got Placebo Be First to Get the Real Thing?," *New York Times*, 3 December 2020, A7.

33 Ibid.

34 WHO Ad Hoc Expert Group on the Next Steps for Covid-19 Vaccine Evaluation, "Placebo-Controlled Trials of Covid-19 Vaccines—Why We Still Need Them," *New England Journal of Medicine* 384 (14 January 2021).

35 Aristotle, *Nicomachean Ethics*, Book I, Chapter 3, in *The Complete Works of Aristotle: The Revised Oxford Translation*, 2 vols., ed. Jonathan Barnes (Princeton, NJ: Princeton University Press, 1984).

36 Gina Kolata, "How a Weighted Lottery Can Offer a Fair Shot," *New York Times*, 23 July 2020; updated 15 December 2020.

37 Robert Wachter and Ashish Jha, "How to Fix the Vaccine Rollout," *New York Times*, 10 January 2021.

38 Kolata, "How a Weighted Lottery."

39 Caroline Chen, "Only Seven of Stanford's First 5,000 Vaccines Were Designated for Medical Residents," *ProPublica*, 18 December 2020.

40 Christine Byers et al., "Doctors Say BJC Prioritizing Older Employees for COVID-19 Vaccine, Not Frontline," *5OnYourSide* (St. Louis), 19 December 2020.

41 Amanda Eisenberg, "Mount Sinai Vaccination of Marketing Staffer Raises Flags at State Health Department," *Politico*, 17 December 2020.

42 Joseph Goldstein, "Hospital Workers Start to 'Turn Against Each Other' to Move Up in Vaccine Line," *New York Times*, 24 December 2020.

43 Mike Petchenik, "Some Metro Atlanta Doctors Concerned about Not Getting Vaccinated against COVID-19 Early Enough," WSB-TV Atlanta, 21 December 2020.

44 Isaac Stanley-Becker and Shawn Boburg, "Wealthy Donors Received Vaccines through Florida Nursing Home," *Washington Post*, 11 January 2021; Gina Bellafante, "How the Wealthy Are Maneuvering to Get the Vaccine First," *New York Times*, 8 January 2021.

45 Lois Taylor, Letter to the Editor, *New York Times*, 8 December 2020.

46 Zeynup Tufekci and Michael Mina, "Maybe Vaccines Can Serve Many More. Let's See," *New York Times*, 19 December 2020; Adrianna Rodriquez, "Debate Over How Many to Vaccinate," *USA Today*, 9 December 2020, D1.

47 Katherine Wu and Rebecca Robbins, "Delay 2nd Doses? Give 2 Half Doses? Vaccine Lag Fuels a Debate," *New York Times*, 5 January 2021, A1.

48 Solarina Ho, "Hiller Asks Canada to Consider Single-Dose Moderna Vaccine, Doctors Skeptical," *CTV News*, 29 December 2020.

49 Andrew MacAskill, "Britain Will Allow Mixing of COVID-19 Vaccines on Rare Occasions," *Reuters*, 2 January 2021.

50 Donald McNeil, "Vaccines Can Be Stretched, but Not Easily," *New York Times*, 2 February 2021, D6.

51 Wu and Robbins, "Delay 2nd Doses?"

52 Ibid.

53 Quoted in Carolyn Johnson, "U.S. Health Officials Say They Plan to Stick with Two-Dose Coronavirus Regimen," *Washington Post*, 4 January 2021.

54 "Study in Israel Shows Pfizer Vaccine 85% Effective after First Dosage: The Lancet," *CNBC News*, 19 February 2021.

55 Apoorva Mandavilli, "People Who Have Had Covid Should Get Just One Dose, Studies Suggest," *New York Times*, 21 February 2021; J. Douglas and M. Colchester, "U.K. Vaccine Data Offer Upbeat Signs," *Wall Street Journal*, 21 February 2021.

56 Carolyn Bormann, "Countdown to Immunity," *New Yorker*, 14 December 2020, 22.

57 Katherine Wu, "Boston Doctor Reports Serious Allergic Reaction after Getting Moderna's Shot," *New York Times*, 25 December 2020.

58 Jop de Vrieze, "Suspicions Grow That Nanoparticles in Pfizer's COVID-19 Vaccine Trigger Rare Allergic Reactions," *Science*, 21 December 2020.

59 Denise Grady et al., "Death of Doctor Who Got Covid Shot Is Investigated," *New York Times*, 13 January 2021.

60 Ibid.

61 Jeremy Strasburg and Joanna Sugden, "Allergic Reactions Seen in 29 in US," *New York Times*, 7 January 2021.

62 Peter Doshi and Jennifer Block, "Don't Pressure the Vaccine Hesitant," *New York Times*, 10 January 2021, SR7.

63 Katherine Wu, "The Second Covid-10 Shot Is a Rude Awakening for Immune Cells," *The Atlantic*, February 2021.

64 Cassandra Willyard, "Survivors Report Intense Side Effects from Vaccine," *New York Times*, 3 February 2021.

65 Scott Gottlieb, "Pharmacies Can Get Shots in Arms," *Wall Street Journal*, 4 January 2021.

66 JoNel Aleccia, "Is Your Covid Vaccine Venue Prepared to Handle Rare, Life-Threatening Reactions?," *Kaiser Health News*, 11 January 2021.

67 Quoted in Donald McNeil, "How Can We Achieve Herd Immunity? Experts Are Quietly Upping the Number," *New York Times*, 24 December 2020.

68 Ibid.

69 Amy Harmon, "They Beat COVID-19, but the Debilitating Effects and Economic Costs May Linger for Years," *Bloomberg News*, 20 August 2020.

70 S. Gupta, "13 People in Israel Suffer Facial Paralysis After Taking Coronavirus Vaccine Shots," *India Times*, 17 January 2021.

71 Noah Weiland et al., "Johnson & Johnson Vaccinations Paused after Rare Clotting Cases Emerge," *New York Times*, 13 April 2021.

72 Daniel Hendandez and Brianna Abbott, "Clotting Disorder Confounds Scientists," *Wall Street Journal*, 14 April 2021, A6.

73 Michael Lederman, Maxwell Mehlman, and Stuart Youngner, "Require Vaccines for All to Defeat COVID," *USA Today*, 10 August 2020, 7A.

74 Anthony Skelton and Lisa Forsberg, "Mandating Vaccination," in *The Ethics of Pandemics*, ed. Meredith Schwartz (Peterborough, ON: Broadview Press, 2020), 131–34.

75 Jared S. Hopkins, "COVID Vaccine Trials Have a Problem: Minority Groups Don't Trust Them," *Wall Street Journal*, 5 August 2020.

76 Kerry Murakami, "Should Students Be Required to Be Vaccinated," *Inside Higher Ed*, 10 July 2020.

77 Ibid.
78 Debbie Kaminer, "Can a Company Mandate Workers to Be Vaccinated," *Birmingham News*, 26 February 2021, C3.
79 L. Gostin et al., "Mandating COVID-19 Vaccines," *Journal of the American Medical Association* 325, no. 6 (29 December 2020): 532–33.
80 Donald McNeil, "Long, Dark Winter before U.S. Gets Vaccines," *New York Times*, 1 December 2020, A10.
81 Ibid.
82 Rebecca Robbins et al., "The Effort to Vaccinate Anxious Medical Workers," *New York Times*, 15 January 2021, D1.
83 Azi Paybarah and Michael Levenson, "Robbins Sued by Employee Who Had Covid," *New York Times*, 26 December 2020.
84 McNeil, "Long, Dark Winter."
85 Noah Weiland, Denise Grady, and David Sanger, "U.S. Places a $2 Billion Wager in the Global Race for a Vaccine," *New York Times*, 22 July 2020.
86 Fraiser Kansteiner, "Pfizer, BioNTech Keep COVID Vaccine Deals Rolling with 120M-Dose Japan Pact," *Fierce Pharma*, 31 July 2020.
87 "Coronavirus Update," *New York Times*, 1 August 2020.
88 Yasmine Hasan "Canada: Is 'Me First' COVID Vaccine Policy Hurting Other Nations?," *Al Jazeera*, 17 December 2020.
89 Megan Twohey et al., "Rush by Rich Countries to Reserve Early Doses Leaves the Poor Behind," *New York Times*, 16 December 2020, A6.
90 Ibid.
91 Ibid.
92 "Should Oxford-AstraZeneca's Progress Worry Moderna?," *Forbes*, 22 July 2020.
93 Quoted in Peter Loftus and Drew Hinshaw, "Countries Vie to Get First Dibs on Vaccine," *Wall Street Journal*, 27 May 2020.
94 Rick Bright, former director of BARDA, was transferred to a meaningless job by President Trump for telling the truth about the lack of readiness in the United States to fight the virus. See ibid.
95 Mueller, "Allies Spar."
96 See https://www.who.int/workforcealliance/members_partners/member_list/gavi/en/.
97 Adam Taylor, "Why Vaccine Nationalism Is Winning," *Washington Post*, 2 September 2020.
98 Richard Engel story on GAVI, *NBC News*, 31 July 2020.
99 Associated Press, "AstraZeneca: No profits from COVID Vaccine," *Tuscaloosa News*, 31 July 2020. Even folks associated with the Oxford vaccine are not angels, and some would profit from a successful vaccine, including Oxford University itself, the two lead scientists, and a private investment firm providing some of the start-up capital. Jenny Strasberg, "Private Investors Stand Ready to Profit from Oxford Vaccine," *Wall Street Journal*, 3 August 2020.
100 Saheed Shah, "Developing Nations Press Vaccine Access," *Wall Street Journal*, 18 November 2020, A8.
101 Peter Loftus, "Drugmakers Start to Signal Prices for Covid-19 Vaccines," *Wall Street Journal*, 5 August 2020.
102 Ibid.
103 Quoted in Elisabetta Povoledo and Marc Santora, "Pope Francis Makes Christmas Appeal for Nations to Share Vaccines," *New York Times*, 25 December 2020.

104 Paul Schemm and Jennifer Hassan, "WHO Chief Warns of 'Catastrophic Moral Failure' as Rich Countries Dominate Vaccine Supplies," *Washington Post*, 18 January 2021.

105 According to WHO Secretary Tedros Ghebreyesus, "'Wall of Inequality': W.H.O. Warns of Vaccine Distribution," *New York Times*, 18 January 2021, A21.

106 "Poll: No Rush in US to Get Vaccine," *USA Today*, 8 September 2020.

107 Loomis, *Epidemics*.

108 Saheed Shah, "Developing Nations Press Vaccine Access," *Wall Street Journal*, 18 November 2020.

109 WHO, "Virtual Symposium to Mark 25 Years of the TRIPS Agreement," https://www.wto.org/english/news_e/news20_e/trip_20nov20_e.htm.

110 E. Urias and S. Ramani, "Access to Medicines after TRIPS: Is Compulsory Licensing an Effective Mechanism to Lower Drug Prices? A Review of the Existing Evidence," *Journal of International Business Policy*, 3 September 2020, 1–18.

111 Ellen 't Hoen et al., "Driving a Decade of Change: HIV/AIDS, Patents and Access to Medicines for All," *Journal of the International AIDS Society* 14, no. 1 (2011): 15.

112 Selam Gebrekidan and Matt Apuzzo, "Missed Chances to Share Doses in Poor Nations," *New York Times*, 22 March 2021, A1.

113 Meghan Twohey and Nicholas Kulish, "Gates' Fortune Looms Large in Mission to Vaccinate World," *New York Times*, 23 November 2020, A1.

114 Thomas Cueni, "The Risk in Suspending Vaccine Patent Rules," *New York Times*, 10 December 2020.

115 James Pooley, "Covid Shakedown at the WTO," *New York Times*, 17 December 2020, A17.

116 Berkeley Lovelace, "Trump Says Coronavirus Vaccine Won't Be Delivered to New York Right Away," *MSNBC*, 13 November 2020.

117 Parisa Hafezi, "Iran Leader Bans Import of U.S., UK COVID-19 Vaccines, Demands Sanctions End," *Reuters*, 9 January 2020.

118 Sui-Lee Wee and Ernesto Londoño, "Disappointing Chinese Vaccine Results Pose Setback for Developing World," *New York Times*, 15 January 2021.

119 Sheryl Gay Stolberg, "Trump Claims Credit for Vaccines. Some of His Backers Don't Want to Take Them," *New York Times*, 19 December 2020, A1.

120 Julie Wernau, "Shot Skeptics Impede Herd Immunity Goal," *Wall Street Journal*, 4 February 2021, A7.

121 Manny Fernandez, "A New Coalition Forms Against Vaccines in California," *New York Times*, 7 February 2021, A6.

122 Mathew Dalton, "Skeptics Mar French Efforts on Vaccination," *Wall Street Journal*, 9 January 2021, A9.

123 Peter Doshi and Jennifer Block, "Don't Pressure the Vaccine Hesitant," *New York Times*, 10 January 2021, SR7.

124 Richard Paddock, "Muslims in Indonesia Ask If Shots are Halal," *New York Times*, 5 January 2021.

125 Elizabeth Dias and Ruth Graham, "White Evangelical Resistance Is Obstacle in Vaccination Push," *New York Times*, 5 April 2021, A1.

126 McNeil, "How Can We Achieve Herd Immunity?"

127 Helen Branswell, "COVID Controversies Webinar: Challenges in COVID Vaccine Allocation & Distribution," Webinar from the University of Minnesota, 8 January 2021.

128 Weise, "50 States, 50 Plans."

129 Editorial, "Avoidable Missteps on Vaccines," *New York Times*, 1 January 2021, A18.

130 Ibid.
131 Elisabeth Rosenthal, "Analysis: Some Said the Vaccine Rollout Would Be a 'Nightmare': They Were Right," *Kaiser Health News*, reprinted in *Miami Herald*, 25 December 2020.
132 Robert Kramer, "Workers Producing the Vaccine Need Vaccination," *Wall Street Journal*, 25 January 2021.
133 Editorial, "In the Dark about the Vaccine Rollout," *New York Times*, 8 February 2021, A22.
134 "EU Vaccine Shortages Snowball into a Crisis," *New York Times*, 12 April 2021.
135 Holman Jenkins, "Vaccines versus Lockdowns," *Wall Street Journal*, 15 December 2020; Meghan Deming et al., "Accelerating Development of SARS Cov-2 Vaccines: The Role for Controlled Human Infection Models," *New England Journal of Medicine*, 3 September 2020.
136 Betsy McKay et al., "Moderna Explores Use of Third Dose," *Wall Street Journal*, 16–17 January 2021, A8.

NOTES TO CHAPTER EIGHT

1 Timothy Chappell, "Two Distinctions that Do Make a Difference: The Action/Omission Distinction and the Principle of Double Effect," *Philosophy* 77, no. 300 (April 2002): 211–33.
2 James Rachels, "Active and Passive Euthanasia," *New England Journal of Medicine* 292 (9 January 1975): 78–80.
3 Philippa Foot, "The Problem of Abortion and the Doctrine of Double Effect," *Oxford Review* 5 (1967); reprinted in Philippa Foot, *Virtues and Vices* (Oxford: Basil Blackwell, 1978).
4 F.M. Kamm, *The Trolley Problem Mysteries* (Oxford: Oxford University Press, 2016), 31.
5 See https://www.youtube.com/watch?v=JWb_svTrcOg.
6 F.M. Kamm, "The Trolley Problem Mysteries," and Judith Thomson, "Kamm on the Trolley Problems," in Kamm, *Trolley Problem Mysteries*.
7 Foot, "The Problem of Abortion."
8 WHO, "Dengue and Severe Dengue," https://www.who.int/news-room/fact-sheets/detail/dengue-and-severe-dengue.
9 Lisa Rosenbaum, "Trolleyology and the Dengue Vaccine Dilemma," *New England Journal of Medicine* 379 (26 July 2018): 305–07.
10 Ibid.
11 Kent Septkowitz, "The 1947 Smallpox Vaccination Campaign in New York City, Revisited," *Emerging Infectious Diseases* 10, no. 5 (May 2004): 960–61. This review undermines some recent claims in the media about the amazing success of this campaign.
12 See Siobhan Roberts, "The Pandemic Is a Prisoner's Dilemma Game," *New York Times*, 20 December 2020.
13 William Poundstone, *Prisoner's Dilemma* (New York: Anchor Books, 1993).
14 Kuhn, Steven, "Prisoner's Dilemma," *The Stanford Encyclopedia of Philosophy*, https://plato.stanford.edu/entries/prisoner-dilemma/.
15 Roberts, "The Pandemic Is a Prisoner's Dilemma Game."
16 Chris T. Bauch, Alison P. Galvani, and David J.D. Earn, "Group Interest versus Self-Interest in Smallpox Vaccination Policy," *Proceedings of the National Academy of Sciences* 100, no. 18 (2 September 2003): 10564–67.

17 Peter Jentsch et al., "Go Big or Go Home: A Model-Based Assessment of General Strategies to Slow the Spread of Forest Pests via Infested Firewood," *PLOS ONE*, 15 September 2020.

18 Sebastian Funk et al., "The Spread of Awareness and Its Impact on Epidemic Outbreaks," *Proceedings of the National Academy of Sciences* 106, no. 16 (21 April 2009): 6872–77.

NOTES TO CHAPTER NINE

1 Alasdair MacIntyre, *A Short History of Ethics* (New York: Macmillan, 1966).

2 See the following works by Michel Foucault: *The Birth of the Clinic: Archaeology of Medical Perception*; *Discipline and Punish: The Birth of the Prison*; *The History of Sexuality*; and *Madness and Civilization: A History of Insanity in the Age of Reason*.

3 See Gregory Pence, *Overcoming Addiction: Seven Imperfect Solutions and the End of America's Greatest Epidemic* (Lanham, MD: Rowman & Littlefield, 2020).

4 Thomas Szasz, *The Myth of Mental Illness* (New York: Harper & Row, 1964).

5 Michel Foucault, *A History of Sexuality*, vols. 1–4, trans. Robert Hurley (New York: Viking, 1986).

6 Christopher Caldwell, "The Coronavirus Philosopher," *New York Times*, 21 August 2020.

7 Thomas Erdbrink, "Dutch Police Clash with Protesters Denouncing Lockdown Measures," *New York Times*, 17 January 2021.

8 Anna Saurbrey, "Germany's Bizarre Lockdown Protests," *New York Times*, 31 August 2020.

9 Matt Ridley, "What the Pandemic Has Taught Us about Science," *Wall Street Journal*, 10–11 October 2020, C1.

10 Robert Nozick, *Anarchy, State and Utopia* (New York: Basic Books, 1974).

11 K.C. Swanson et al., "Contact Tracing Performance during the Ebola Epidemic in Liberia, 2014–2015," *PLOS Neglected Tropical Diseases* 12, no. 9 (2018).

12 Sara Otterman, "They Praised Contact Tracing Rollout: Workers Called It Chaos," *New York Times*, 29 July 2020.

13 Jake Selner, "Cardinals Contact Tracer Finds 'Tricky' Balance," *Associated Press*, 1 August 2020.

14 Deanna Paul, "Delays in Test Results Cost Workers," *Wall Street Journal*, 3 August 2020, A6.

15 Otterman, "They Praised Contact Tracing Rollout."

16 Ibid.

17 Ed Shanahan, "It Took Subpoenas for 8 Partygoers to Work with Investigators in New York Suburb," *New York Times*, 7 August 2020.

18 "News of the 50+ States: Connecticut," *USA TODAY*, 4 August 2020, 5D.

19 Matt Richtel, "Emerging Tools Make Contact Tracing Easier, but All Have Tradeoffs," *New York Times*, 3 June 2020; updated 28 January 2021.

20 Wright, "The Plague Year."

21 Richtel, "Emerging Tools."

22 Peer Hessler, "The Sealed City," *New Yorker*, 12 October 2020, 40.

23 Catherine Porter, "Covid Shaming, Virulent in Canada, Caused Him to Flee Town," *New York Times*, 22 February 2021.

24 Peggy Noonan, "The Challenge of Contact Tracing in America," *Wall Street Journal*, 30-31 May 2020, A13.

25 Jennifer Steinhauer and Abby Goodnough, "Contact Tracing Has Largely Failed in the U.S.," *New York Times*, 1 August 2020, A1.

26 David Thomas et al., "Genetic Variation in *IL28B* and Spontaneous Clearance of Hepatitis C Virus," *Nature* 461, no. 7265 (8 October 2009): 798–801.

27 Arthur Caplan, "Are COVID-19 Swab Samples a Threat to Your DNA Privacy?" *MEDSCAPE*, 13 January 2021.

NOTES TO CHAPTER TEN

1   Alicia Widge et al., "Durability of Responses after SARS-CoV-2 mRNA-1273 Vaccination," *New England Journal of Medicine* 384 (7 January 2021): 80–82.

2   Quoted by Stacey McKenna, "Vaccines Need Not Completely Stop COVID Transmission to Curb the Pandemic," *Scientific American*, 21 January 2021.

3   Megan Marples, "When Should You Get the Vaccine If You Have Had Covid-19? Dr. Wen Explains," *CNN Health*, 11 April 2021.

4   Centers for Disease Control, "Frequently Asked Questions about COVID-19 Vaccination," 28 December 2020; updated 12 March 2021, https://www.cdc.gov/coronavirus/2019-ncov/vaccines/faq.html.

5   Peter Loftus, "Vaccine Study on Campuses Held Up," *Wall Street Journal*, 4 January 2021.

6   Samantha Pearson et al., "Brazil Launches Key Vaccine Test," *Wall Street Journal*, 18 February 2021, A9.

7   Sridhar Chilmuri, comment on Siri R. Kadire, Robert M. Wachter, and Nicole Lurie, "Delayed Second Dose versus Standard Regimen for Covid-19 Vaccination," *New England Journal of Medicine*, 19 February 2021.

8   Sumathi Reddy, "Can You Still Spread the Virus after Vaccination?" *Wall Street Journal*, 12 January 2021, A12.

9   Charles Toutant, "People Are Now Suing Their Bosses over COVID-19 at Work, but Can They Win in Court?," Law.com, 3 November 2020.

10 Scott McCartney, "The Airlines Bet on Covid Tests," *Wall Street Journal*, 17 December 2020, A11.

11 Maria Cramer, "Fights and 'Mob Mentality': What Flight Attendants Faced over the Last Year," *New York Times* (1 February 2021).

12 Françoise Baylis and Natalie Kofler, "COVID Immunity Testing: A Passport to Inequity," *Issues in Science and Technology*, 29 April 2020.

13 *BBC News*, 28 December 2020.

14 See Rapid Acceleration of Diagnostics (RADX), https://www.nih.gov/research-training/medical-research-initiatives/radx.

15 Alyson Krueger, "New Velvet Rope: Rapid Tests," *New York Times*, 16 August 2020, D1, D8.

16 Ibid., D8.

17 Jonah Engel Bromwich, "For Some, A Shot above the Rest," *New York Times*, 24 January 2021, D6.

18 Kwame Anthony Appiah, *Cosmopolitanism: Ethics in a World of Strangers* (New York: Norton, 2006).

19 Garrett Hardin, *Exploring New Ethics for Survival: The Voyage of the Spaceship Beagle* (New York: Pelican, 1973).

20 Bobbie Farsides, "The Troubling Prospect of Immunity Certificates," Nuffield Council on Bioethics, webinar, 9 July 2020.

21 Ibid.

22 Ibid.

23 Alexandra Phelan, "COVID-19 Immunity Passports and Vaccination Certificates: Scientific, Equitable, and Legal Challenges," *The Lancet*, 4 May 2020, 1595–98.

24 Rebecca Brown, Dominic Kelly, Dominic Wilkinson, and Julian Savulescu, "The Scientific and Ethical Feasibility of Immunity Passports," *The Lancet: Infectious Diseases*, 16 October 2020, e58–e63.

25 Ibid., e61.

26 The main story was reported at a city council meeting in Tuscaloosa, Alabama, home of the original campus of the University of Alabama, and was told by a councilman who heard from a local doctor who ran a testing site for Covid out of his Urgent Care Center. A person called one day to find his results and who sounded like a student and who, the physician believed, seemed happy to get a positive result. On the basis of that call, the physician inferred that the student had been a member of a group, possibly a fraternity, that had deliberately tried to get infected. No follow-up or evidence for this inference was ever presented, although the story made national and international news.

27 E. Levinson, "Yes, You Can Still Get Infected with COVID-19 after Being Vaccinated. Here's Why," *CTV News*, 8 January 2021.

28 CDC, "Post Vaccine Considerations for Healthcare Personnel," updated 13 December 2020, https://www.cdc.gov/coronavirus/2019-ncov/hcp/post-vaccine-consider ations-healthcare-personnel.html.

29 William A. Haseltine, "Israeli Study Shows a Majority of Those Vaccinated Can Be Infected by SARS-CoV-2 after the First Shot," *Forbes*, 27 January 2021.

30 Benedict Carey, "One Flight, Multiple Infections: A Clear Warning," *New York Times*, 12 January 2021, D5.

31 Krueger, "New Velvet Rope," D8.

32 Fauci, "Fauci to Medscape."

33 S.F. Lumley et al., "Antibody Status and Incidence of SARS-COV-2 Infection in Health Care Workers," *New England Journal of Medicine* 384 (11 February 2021): 533–40.

34 Former CDC director Thomas Frieden, *CBS Morning Show*, 23 December 2020.

35 "Mass Vaccination: Questions over Safety and Who Gets a Shot as Inoculations Begin," *New York Times*, 9 December 2020, A9.

36 Benjamin Katz, "Airlines, EU Split on Implementing Vaccine Passports," *Wall Street Journal*, 5 April 2021, A9; Saskia Popescu and Alexandra Phelan, "Vaccine Passports Are No Panacea," *New York Times*, 26 March 2021, A26.

37 Sheera Frenkel, "Forged Proof of Vaccines Litters Web," *New York Times*, 9 April 2021, A1.

38 Benjamin Katz, "Airlines Struggle to Police Falsified Covid-19 Papers," *Wall Street Journal*, 14 April 2021, A6.

39 Christopher Elliott, "Proof of Vaccination Looms as a Travel Issue in Pandemic World," *Washington Post*, 23 January 2021.

40 CDC, "Requirement for Proof of Negative COVID-19 Test or Recovery from COVID-19 for All Air Passengers Arriving in the United States," updated 2 March 2021, https://www.cdc.gov/coronavirus/2019-ncov/travelers/testing-international-air-travelers.html.

NOTES TO CHAPTER ELEVEN

1 Paul Farmer, "Rethinking Medical Ethics: A View from Below," *Developing World Bioethics* 4, no. 1 (May 2004).
2 Homer Venters, former chief medical officer at New York City's Riker Island jail complex, quoted in "1 in 5 State, Federal Prisoners Has Had the Coronavirus," *Associated Press*, 20 December 2020.
3 Troy Closson, "Hard Hit by Virus, New York Inmates Are Left Off Vaccine Plan," *New York Times*, 26 January 2021.
4 Jordan Culver, "1K Cases and Counting at San Quentin Prison," *USA Today*, 15 July 2020.
5 Jennifer Steinhauer and Thomas Neff, "At Local Bases and Overseas, the Military Is Awash in Coronavirus Cases," *New York Times*, 23 July 2020.
6 "COVID-19: Law Enforcement Deaths," *Police1*, 28 January 2021.
7 Sky Chadde, "Tracking COVID-19's Impact on Meatpacking Workers and Industry," Midwest Center for Covid-19 Tracking, 16 April 2020, https://investigatemidwest.org/2020/04/16/tracking-covid-19s-impact-on-meatpacking-workers-and-industry/.
8 Christina Jewett, "More Than 2,900 Health Care Workers Died This Year—And the Government Barely Kept Track," *KLN News*, 23 December 2020.
9 Apoorva Mandavilli, "Scientists Urge D.D.C. for Air Workplace Mandates, Now," *New York Times*, 18 February 2021.
10 Jamie Ducharme and Elijah Wolfson, "Does ZIP Code Equal Life Expectancy?" *Time*, 8 July 2019, 8.
11 David Goodman, "Two Neighborhoods: One Rich, One Poor, One Spared," *New York Times*, 22 July 2020, A6.
12 Mini Kagi, "300,000 Seafarers Still Stuck on Ships: 'We Feel Like Hostages,'" *ABC News*, 11 September 2020; "Crews Stuck at Sea as Companies Plan for Restart," *Miami Herald*, 18 November 2020.
13 Jill Cowan, "Why Long Beach Is a Model for the Vaccine Rollout," *New York Times*, 3 February 2021.
14 Alexandra Olson, "Only 13 States Let Grocery Workers Sign Up for Vaccines," *Associated Press*, 20 February 2021.
15 Quoted in Jon Kamp, "Elderly Get A Big Boost from Shots," *Wall Street Journal*, 27–28 March 2021, A6.
16 Michele K. Evans, "Covid's Color Line—Infectious Disease, Inequity, and Racial Justice," *New England Journal of Medicine* 383 (30 July 2020): 5; Jayme Frasier et al., "Why Latinos Suffered Worst Hit," *USA Today*, 30 July 2020, 1-3A.
17 Susan Driggers, "Fouad, Ruffin and Vickers: COVID Is Disproportionately High in African Americans," *UAB News*, 17 July 2020.
18 Katherine Wu, "The Puzzle of Obesity and COVID-19," *New York Times*, 29 September 2020.
19 CDC, "Body Mass Index and Risks of COVID-19," 8 March 2021, https://www.cdc.gov/mmwr/volumes/70/wr/mm7010e4.htm.
20 Gina Kolata, "Americans Blame Obesity on Willpower, Despite Evidence It's Genetic," *New York Times*, 1 November 2016, A1.
21 Charles M. Blow, "Social Distancing Is a Privilege," *New York Times*, 6 April 2020, A23.
22 "News of the 50 States+: Mississippi," *USA Today*, 6 August 2020, 5D.
23 Heather Kovich, "Rural Matters: Coronavirus and the Navajo Nation," *New England Journal of Medicine* 383 (9 July 2020): 2.

24 G.A. Bilkey et al., "Optimizing Precision Medicine for Public Health," *Front Public Health*, 7 March 2019; W. Kalow, "Pharmacogenetics and Pharmacogenomics: Origin, Status, and the Hope for Personalized Medicine," *Pharmacogenomics Journal* 6, no. 3 (2006): 162–65.

25 Ross Douthat, "When You Can't Just 'Trust the Science,'" *New York Times*, 19 December 2020.

26 Kathleen Page and Alejandra Flores-Miller, "Lessons We've Learned: Covid-19 and the Undocumented Latinx Community," *New England Journal of Medicine* 384 (7 January 2021): 1.

27 Jeneen Interlandi, "The Coronavirus Race Gap Explained," *New York Times*, 4 October 2020, SR4.

28 Douthat, "When You Can't Just 'Trust the Science.'"

29 Sarah Whites-Koditschek, "Low Income Blacks, Latinos, Skeptical," *Birmingham News*, 17 January 2021, A9.

30 Audrey Kearney et al., "Attitudes towards COVID-19 Vaccination among Black Women and Men," Kaiser Family Foundation, 19 February 2021.

31 Tonyaa Weatherbee, "Vaccine Trust Low for Black People," *USA Today*, 17 December 2020, D1.

32 Julie Wernau, "Some Health Workers Shun Vaccines," *Wall Street Journal*, 1 February 2021, A7.

33 Isabella Kwai, "Concern in UK Grows as Minority Groups Balk at Covid Inoculation," *New York Times*, 26 January 2021, A9.

34 Charles M. Blow, "How Black People Learned Not to Trust," *New York Times*, 6 December 2020.

35 Jared S. Hopkins, "COVID Vaccine Trials Have a Problem: Minority Groups Don't Trust Them," *Wall Street Journal*, 5 August 2020.

36 Marco Della Cava, Daniel Gonzalez, and Rebecca Plevin, "Undocumented Immigrants Fear Getting Vaccines," *USA Today*, 19 December 2020, D1, D3.

37 Interlandi, "The Coronavirus Race Gap Explained."

38 Erica Green, "Surge of Suicides Forces Las Vegas Schools to Reopen," *New York Times*, 24 January 2021.

39 Alexa Norton, "Applying the Lessons of COVID-19 Response to Canada's Worsening Opioid Epidemic," *EClinical Medicine* 29 (1 December 2020): 100633.

40 David Brooks, "Children Need to Be Back in School Now," *New York Times*, 30 January 2021, A23.

NOTES TO CHAPTER TWELVE

1 Plato, *Republic*, in *The Collected Dialogues of Plato*, trans. Paul Shorey, ed. E. Hamilton and H. Cairns (Princeton, NJ: Princeton University Press, 1961), 601 (351d).

2 Spinney, "What Does the Spanish Flu of 1918 Teach Us?"

3 Jared Diamond, *Guns, Germs and Steel*, and *Collapse: How Societies Choose to Fail or Succeed* (New York: Norton, 1999).

4 For more on these distinctions, see Gregory E. Pence, "Recent Work on the Virtues," *American Philosophical Quarterly* 21, no. 4 (1984): 281–97.

5 Wright, "The Plague Year," 22.

6 Ibid.

7 Matt Apuzzo et al., "How the World Missed COVID's Symptom-Free Carriers," *New York Times*, 23 July 2020, A1, A10.

8   Marr, "Yes, the Coronavirus Is in the Air."

9   Drew Hinshaw and Betsy McKay, "WHO Faults Itself Over Outbreak," *Wall Street Journal*, 13 May 2021, A9.

10 "News from the Newsroom: Overnight Emails Tell the Story of 2020," *New York Times*, 3 January 2021, 2.

11 Bob Woodward, *Rage* (New York: Simon & Schuster, 2020), xix-xx.

12 Lew Serviss and Azi Paybarah, "'One Day—It's like a Miracle—It Will Disappear: What Trump Said about the Pandemic and Masks," *New York Times*, 2 October 2020.

13 Michael Bender and Rebbeca Ballhaus, "'Try Getting It Yourselves': Trump Sowed Pandemic Supply Chaos," *Wall Street Journal*, 1 September 2020, A1, A10.

14 "Coronavirus: Outcry after Trump Suggests Injecting Disinfectant as Treatment," *BBC News*, 24 April 2020.

15 Michael Shear et al., "President's Focus in the Management of the Pandemic: Himself," *New York Times*, 1 January 2021.

16 Editorial Board, USA Today, "100,000 Coronavirus Deaths Mark an American Tragedy," *USA Today*, 27 May 2020.

17 Christine Cabera, "Trump Falsely Claims COVID-19 Is 'Dying Out' as Cases Surge in Over 20 States," *TPM*, 18 June 2020.

18 Shear et al., "President's Focus."

19 Quoted by Nicholas Kristoff, "A Colossal Failure of Leadership," *New York Times*, 25 October 2020.

20 Ashley Coleman, "The Rise and Fall of White House COVID-19 Advisor Dr. Scott Atlas...," *Business Insider*, 1 December 2020.

21 Chris Buckley, "China's Nationalists Sneer at US Troubles," *New York Times*, 14 December 2020.

22 Li Yuan, "Freedom Through a Chinese Looking Glass," *New York Times*, 5 January 2021, B1, B6.

23 Aylin Woodward, "A New Documentary Shows How a Top CDC Official Who Warned Americans about the Coronavirus Promptly Vanished from Public View," *Business Insider*, 20 October 2020.

24 Kristen Holmes et al., "Whistleblower: US Workers Not Protected When Greeting Coronavirus Evacuees at California Military Bases," *Mercury News*, 27 February 2020.

25 Sheryl Gay Stolberg, "Trump Administration to Collect Hospital's Virus Data from Now On," *New York Times*, 15 July 2020.

26 Apoorva Mandavilli, "CDC Finds Big Differences in Infections vs. Reported Cases," *New York Times*, 22 July 2020.

27 Adriana Rodriguez, "Children Get Milder Cases, Can Be Carriers," *USA Today*, 12 July 2020.

28 Alex Woodward, "Coronavirus: US Surgeon General Admits He Shouldn't Have Compared Virus to the Flu," *The Independent*, 6 April 2020.

29 Jordan Fischer, "Hogan: Maryland National Guard Protecting Coronavirus Tests to Stop Feds from Taking Them," *WUSA /9News*, 30 April 2020.

30 Ibid.

31 Alan Brandt and Alyssa Botelho, "Not a Perfect Storm: COVID and the Importance of Language," *New England Journal of Medicine* 382 (16 April 2020): 1493-95.

32 Tom Avril, "Study: Next Coronavirus May Already Be Circulating in Bats," *Philadelphia Inquirer*, 8 August 2020, reprinted in *Tuscaloosa News*, 9 August 2020.

33 Katie Rogers et al., "Trump Calls it 'Chinese Virus'...," *New York Times*, 18 March 2020.

34 Nicholas Fandos, "Anti-Mask Louie Gohmert Tests Positive, Sending Shudders through Congress,' *New York Times*, 29 July 2020.

35 Kimmy Yam, "There Were 3,800 Anti-Asian Racist Incidents, Mostly against Women, in Past Year," *NBC News*, 21 March 2021.

36 Richard Wike, J. Fetterholf, and M. Mordecai, "U.S. Image Plummets Internationally as Most Say Country Has Handled Coronavirus Badly," *Reuters*, September 2020.

37 Marine Strauss, "China's Response to COVID-19 Better Than U.S.'s, Global Poll Finds," *Reuters*, 15 June 2020.

38 Hanna Beech, "'I Feel Sorry for Americans': U.S. Tumult Baffles the World," *New York Times*, 26 September 2020, A7.

39 Li Yuan, "Freedom through a Chinese Looking Glass," *New York Times*, 4 January 2020, B1, B6.

40 Wike et al., "U.S. Image Plummets Internationally."

41 Michael Baker and Andrew Anglemyer, "Successful Elimination of COVID Transmission in New Zealand," *New England Journal of Medicine* 383 (7 August 2020).

42 Anthony Fauci, interviewed on ABC's *Good Morning America*, 2 February 2021.

NOTES TO CHAPTER THIRTEEN

1 Michael Osterholm, "Three Possible Waves," https://www.businessinsider.com/coronavirus-pandemic-could-last-2-years-resurge-in-fall-2020-5?r=US&IR=T.

2 Siobhan Roberts, "How Will Distant Waves of Infection Break?" *New York Times*, 8 May 2020.

3 Quoted by Daniel Hernandez and Drew Hinshaw, "Virus Likely to Stay after Crisis Fades," *Wall Street Journal*, 8 February 2021, A1, A6.

4 Max Colchester and Jason Douglas, "Gains in Vaccines Mask Sobering Truths," *Wall Street Journal*, 23 February 2021.

5 Devi Sridhar, "GPS with Fareed Zakaria," CNN, 6 March 2021.

6 Berkeley Lovelace Jr., "Pfizer CEO Says Third Covid Vaccine Dose Likely Needed within 12 Months," *CNBC News*, 15 April 2021.

7 Quoted in Drew Hinshaw and Joanna Sugden, "Slow Vaccine Roll Out Puts Crimp in Plans," *Wall Street Journal*, 13 December 2020, A7.

8 CDC, CDC COVID Data Tracker: Variant Proportions, 10 April 2021.

9 CDC, "COVID-19 Breakthrough Case Investigations and Reporting," https://www.cdc.gov/vaccines/covid-19/health-departments/breakthrough-cases.html.

10 L. Gostin et al., "Mandating COVID-19 Vaccines," *Journal of the American Medical Association* 325, no. 6 (29 December 2020): 532–33.

11 Matthew Haag, "Waitress Says Refusal to Get Shot Was Behind Her Firing by Restaurant," *New York Times*, 18 February 2021, A8.

12 Alex de Waal and Paul Richards, "Coronavirus: Why Lockdowns May Not Be the Answer in Africa," *BBC News*, 14 April 2020.

13 Sridhar, "GPS with Fareed Zakaria."

14 Greg Ip, "Post-Covid Recovery Divides Rich Nations from Poor," *Wall Street Journal*, 19 January 2021, R1, R8.

15 Quoted by Frank Bruni, "Years of Death and Rage," *New York Times*, 3 May 2020, 7.

16 Jonah Engel Bromwich, "For Some, a Shot above the Rest," *New York Times*, 16 January 2021, D6.

17 Andrew Jacobs, "One Year In, Pandemic Pushes Health Care Workers to the Brink," *New York Times*, 5 February 2021, A6.

18 Drew Hinshaw, "WHO Faulted for Virus Response," *Wall Street Journal*, 20 January 2021, A9.
19 Betsy McKay and Drew Hinshaw, "The WHO's Flawed Design Was No Match for Covid," *Wall Street Journal*, 29–30 August 2020, A1, A10.
20 Ibid.
21 Betsy McKay, "New CDC Director Pledges to Restore Trust," *Wall Street Journal*, 20 January 2021, A3.
22 Donald McNeil and Thomas Kaplan, "US Will Rejoin Global Virus-Hunting Effort that Ended Last Year," *New York Times*, 31 August 2020, A4.
23 Tom Frieden, "Will We Ready for the Next Pandemic?," *Wall Street Journal*, 13 February 2021.
24 Sources differ about how many jobs were scrapped. Michael Sparer, "We Need a Voice for Public Health," *New York Times*, 29 May 2020, says 56,000, but a survey by Kaiser Health News and the Associated Press said 38,000: Lauren Weber, "Pandemic Backlash Jeopardizes Public Health," *KHN*, 20 December 2020.
25 Sparer, "We Need a Voice."
26 Nicholas Kristoff, "2 Scenarios for Covid-19: Best and Worst," *New York Times*, 20 March 2020.
27 Lisa Winter, "Conference Linked to as Many as 300,000 Covid-19 Cases: Study," *The Scientist*, 14 December 2020.
28 Steven Lee Myers, "Facing Fresh Flare-Ups, China Puts More Than 22 Million on Lockdown," *New York Times*, 14 January 2021.
29 Julie Bykowicz, "Virus Deepens a Divide in Pennsylvania," *Wall Street Journal*, 10 February 2021, A6.
30 J. Gettelman et al., "India's Latest Covid Wave is Disturbingly Different," *New York Times*, 29 April 2021, A6; Shan Li, "'Double Mutant' Variant Hits India Hard," *Wall Street Journal*, 24-25 April 2021, A7.
31 "Vaccine Can Turn People Into Crocodiles," *Hindu Times*, 20 December 2020.
32 Brilliant et al., "Herd Immunity Won't Save Us."
33 "World Population by Year," *Worldometer*. https://www.worldometers.info/world population/world-population-by-year/.

ACKNOWLEDGMENTS

Many people helped me research and write this book. Dennis Watts, retired professor of medicine from UAB, critiqued every chapter and fed me voluminous citations every day. Independent philosopher Alfred N. Garwood also critiqued every chapter and sent me material. Immunology majors Joy Duan and Kristine Farag proved especially skillful as fact-checkers. Bioethics major Annalise van der Wel used her excellent proofing and editing skills to tighten the writing. Connie Shao, a surgical resident at UAB, read chapters of the manuscript for sense. My old study partner from William & Mary, Bert Lindler, a journalist and Neiman fellow at Harvard, also checked and critiqued chapters, as did my brother-in-law, Dave Kummerlowe. Anna Townsend, Ritika Samant, Alp Turgut, and Mel Ebeling helped research specific topics. Canadian Charlene Mansour helped research Covid in Canada. Historian Michael Flannery used early chapters in his honors seminar at UAB and allowed me to vet them with his class.

I am especially indebted to my wife Pat, who carefully read every line of the book and made it clearer, more factual, and more grammatical.

I also learned by serving on UAB's campus vaccine committee, working with my former medical students Sarah Nafziger, head of vaccine distribution for UAB and central Alabama, and Paul Erwin, now Dean of Public Health at UAB. Philosophy chair David Chan sent me key early articles; Provost Pam Benoit supported special lectures on Covid. My weekly walks with retired philosophy professor G. Lynn Stephens led me to read new books and refine my ideas. Lynn also read the penultimate version and saved me from some historical mistakes. My teaching assistant in the summer of 2020 and spring of 2021, Carly Snidow, read and proofed each chapter.

In the summers of 2020 and 2021, I was privileged to teach a graduate seminar in pandemic bioethics in the Global Master's program at UAB, a live Zoom course with students from across North America and the globe. Thanks to Dean Paul Erwin for setting this up. These students, practicing public health and dealing with SARS2 daily, added greatly to my knowledge.

Over the last 45 years, I have been privileged to teach thousands of medical students at UAB, several hundred of whom I began to know as their mentor in our Early Medical School Acceptance Program (EMSAP). I am lucky to still be in contact with so many of them, and they keep me honest and knowledgeable about life in our Covid world for those on the front lines. During this pandemic, they and their families have borne an awful burden, and sometimes with a horrible lack of national support, but they have risen to the test, for which America should be more grateful. I also thank ESMAP students Tanvee Sinha, Alp Turgut, and Nikhita Mudium for proofing this book.

Broadview Press and editor Stephen Latta have been wonderful: efficient, supportive, and highly professional. Stephen's suggestions tweaking the book's organization and adding more material about Canada were extremely helpful. Martin Boyne was superbly professional and the best copy editor with whom I've had the privilege to work. Joe Davies proofed the final version and saved me from many minor mistakes. All in all, I could not have found a better publisher for this book.

ABOUT THE AUTHOR

Gregory Pence first published in bioethics in 1972 as a graduate student at New York University. At the University of Alabama at Birmingham (UAB), he taught for 33 years a required course in medical ethics to 165 medical students and served for 22 years as bioethicist on its Institutional Review Board, reviewing one of the biggest caseloads in the United States. In the 1980s, he served on two AIDS committees at UAB and became Chair of the Board of Birmingham AIDS Outreach, the largest organization in Alabama serving HIV+ people.

He is known for his writings on human cloning; in 2001, he testified against criminalization of all forms of human cloning before committees of the US Congress and the California Senate. His text, *Medical Ethics*, enjoys its 30th year with McGraw-Hill. He has published 8 trade books, edited 4 others, and penned over 70 op-ed essays, which can be found at gregorypence.net.

At UAB, he chaired the philosophy department for six years; still directs the Early Medical School Acceptance Program (EMSAP); won the President's Award for Excellence in Teaching, the Ingalls Award for Distinction in Lifetime Teaching, and the Ireland Award for Distinguished Scholarship; and, most recently, advised the UAB campus committee overseeing distribution of vaccines against Covid.

INDEX